NIGHTMARE

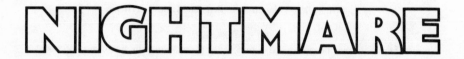

NIGHTMARE

WOMEN AND THE DALKON SHIELD

Susan Perry and Jim Dawson

MACMILLAN PUBLISHING COMPANY
New York

Library of Congress Cataloging-in-Publication Data
Perry, Susan.
Nightmare : Women and the Dalkon Shield.
1. A. H. Robins Company.   2. Dalkon Shield
(Intrauterine contraceptive).   3. Intrauterine
contraceptives—Complications and sequelae.
4. Intrauterine contraceptives industry—United
States.   I. Dawson, Jim (James L.).   II. Title.
HD9995.C64A236   1985   338.7′616139435   85-13710
ISBN 0-02-595930-1

MACMILLAN PUBLISHING COMPANY
866 Third Avenue, New York, N.Y. 10022
Collier Macmillan Canada, Inc.

Macmillan books are available at special discounts for bulk purchases for sales promotions, premiums, fund-raising, or educational use. For details, contact:
Special Sales Director
Macmillan Publishing Company
866 Third Avenue
New York, N.Y. 10022

10 9 8 7 6 5 4 3 2 1

Printed in the United States of America

to Erin and Dylan

Contents

CONTENTS

Introduction and Acknowledgments

W e first met Cynthia Parker in the corridor outside a federal courtroom in Minneapolis on February 29, 1984. Although it was an unseasonably warm day, she clutched her arms to her body, as if chilled. She had never talked to a journalist before—or even been in a courtroom—so she was a little nervous, she explained. She looked around her at the groups of lawyers huddled in various corners of the corridor, small enclaves of dark suits and solemn faces. She said she had no real idea of what was going on here this morning, but had felt a need to come, to see the people who had caused her so much sadness. She had hoped for the chance to speak in court, but it didn't look as though she would get that chance now. Still, she wanted to tell her story to someone. She paused and took a deep breath as if preparing herself for the pain the telling would bring.

Then, in a steady, clear voice, she began to tell of an intrauterine device that had brought tragedy to her life. Her story was similar to the stories of thousands of women, women who had suffered spontaneous abortions, perforated uteri, infections, sterility, and even death after placing their trust in this new, modern contraceptive. We were to hear many of these stories in the months to come.

Cynthia was crying when she finished telling her story. She turned to a group of men huddled a few yards down the corridor. "I really wish I could tell them face to face what they did to me and my family. But they have such a wall up around them psychologically and legally," she said.

A buzzer sounded, indicating that the court recess was over. The men near Cyndi quickly broke up their circle and filed into the courtroom. They were the executives and lawyers of the A. H. Robins Company, the makers of the Dalkon Shield, the IUD that had so altered Cynthia's life.

Cynthia was right about the wall. For 14 years, the executives of the A. H. Robins Company had carefully insulated themselves from the pain and tragedy of so many of the women who had used the Dalkon Shield. But it was a wall that was about to crack.

After she returned to her seat in the back of the courtroom, Cynthia witnessed one of the most dramatic speeches ever directed at corporate executives by a federal judge. U.S. District Judge Miles Lord harshly chastised the A. H. Robins executives, charging that they had caused "monstrous mischief" by marketing a defective and dangerous contraceptive device to millions of women. It was a speech that quickly brought the judge to national attention; Lord became a hero to those who have long fought against corporate indifference and irresponsibility.

But the true heroines in the Dalkon Shield story are women like Cynthia Parker, women who, as Lord said in his speech, "gave up part of their womanhood" so that the A. H. Robins Company might prosper. Yet that afternoon in Lord's courtroom Cynthia sat unnoticed by the press. Lord's speech had been delivered on behalf of women like her, yet as happens so frequently, the individual victims in a tragedy recede into the background as lawyers, bureaucrats, politicians, corporate officials, and others emerge to battle each other.

This book attempts to tell the story of the Dalkon Shield from what we believe is its proper perspective—the perspective of the thousands of women who suffered because they wore small, white, crab-shaped IUDs. in their uteri.

For this is a story that could only have happened to women. As Lord himself said, "I dread to think what would have been the consequences if your victims had been men rather than women, women who seem through some strange quirk of our society's mores to be expected to suffer pain, shame, and humiliation."

This is a book about those women, and for those women.

Many people helped make this book possible. Most of all, we want to thank the courageous women who relived their often painful experiences with the Dalkon Shield for us, especially the women whose stories are recounted within these pages: Pam Van Duyn, Linda Towle, Peggy Mample, Cynthia Parker, and Connie Deemer.

Many others patiently assisted us with many aspects of this book. We would like to especially thank Michael Ciresi, Roger Brosnahan, Michele Bartoli, Jane Fantel, Michael Pretl, Bob Erwin, Patricia Hartmann, and Paula Maccabee. Thanks also to the Women's Health Network, which has been one of the most vocal advocates for Dalkon Shield victims. And our very special thanks to Bob Olson.

We would also like to acknowledge those past and present A. H. Robins officials and attorneys who discussed with us their perspective of the Dalkon Shield story: William Zimmer, William Forrest, Dr. Jack Freund, Dr. Fletcher Owen, and Alexander Slaughter.

Our deepest gratitude to Heide Lange, who from the beginning shared our enthusiasm for this project, and to Alexia Dorszynski, for her editorial guidance and unwavering commitment to the book.

Finally, we wish to thank Juanita Bernard, whose loving care of our children made the writing of this book possible.

Cast of Characters

GRIFFIN BELL: former attorney general of the United States under President Jimmy Carter who represented A. H. Robins in Judge Miles Lord's misconduct hearing

ERNEST BENDER: vice-president, administrative staff, A. H. Robins, 1970; senior vice-president, administrative and corporate planning, A. H. Robins, 1975–1979

ANNE BOARD, M.D.: physician who worked in A. H. Robins' medical services department

JOHN BOARD, M.D.: obstetrician-gynecologist at the Medical College of Virginia and consultant to A. H. Robins

ROGER BROSNAHAN: attorney with the Minnesota law firm of Robins, Zelle, Larson, and Kaplan

JOHN BURKE: general sales manager, A. H. Robins, 1970–1973; vice-president, sales, 1973

DONALD CHRISTIAN, M.D.: head of the obstetrics-gynecology department at the University of Arizona Medical Center and author of an article published in the June 1974 *American Journal of Obstetrics & Gynecology* that reported the connection between septic abortion and the Dalkon Shield

MICHAEL CIRESI: attorney with the Minnesota law firm of Robins, Zelle, Larson, and Kaplan

FRED CLARK, M.D.: A. H. Robins medical director

RAMSEY CLARK: attorney general under President Lyndon Johnson who represented Judge Miles Lord against charges of judicial misconduct brought by A. H. Robins

ROBERT COHN: Connecticut attorney and friend of Irwin Lerner who was one of the original three stockholders in the Dalkon Corporation

WAYNE CROWDER: quality control supervisor, Chap Stick Company, 1968–1978

HUGH DAVIS, M.D.: co-inventor with Irwin Lerner of the Dalkon Shield

CONNIE DEEMER: Wichita woman who in 1975 won the first Dalkon Shield case against A. H. Robins

RICHARD DICKEY, M.D.: associate professor of obstetrics-gynecology at Louisiana State University School of Medicine and member of the FDA's Device Panel

THAD EARL, M.D.: general practitioner from Defiance, Ohio, who bought an interest in the Dalkon Corporation to become its fourth stockholder and its medical director

MARION FINKEL: deputy director of the Bureau of Drugs, FDA

L. H. FOUNTAIN: Democratic Representative from North Carolina who chaired the 1973 "Fountain Hearings" on IUDs

WILLIAM FORREST: secretary and general counsel, A. H. Robins, 1970; vice-president, 1974

DANIEL FRENCH: president, Chap Stick Company

JACK FREUND, M.D.: vice-president of A. H. Robins' medical department, 1970; later, senior vice-president

EMMANUEL FRIEDMAN, M.D.: physician who resigned in protest from the FDA's Device Panel when the FDA decided to end the moratorium on the Shield

DELPHIS GOLDBERG: consultant to the House Intergovernmental Relations Subcommittee during the 1973 "Fountain Hearings" on IUDs

GILBERT GOLDHAMMER: consultant to the House Intergovernmental Relations Subcommittee during the 1973 "Fountain Hearings" on IUDs

WILLIAM GOODRICH: attorney for the FDA

ERNST GRAFENBERG, M.D.: German gynecologist and inventor of the Grafenberg Ring; the man generally regarded as the "father of the IUD"

PETER HUTT: attorney for the FDA

EDMUND JONES: employee of the Ortho Pharmaceutical Company and co-inventor with Hugh Davis of the INCON, the IUD prototype for the Dalkon Shield

OSCAR KLIOZE: director of A. H. Robins' pharmaceutical research and analytical services division

PATRICIA LASHLEY: William Forrest's secretary; later, his paralegal assistant, A. H. Robins

IRWIN "WIN" LERNER: Connecticut engineer who co-invented the Dalkon Shield with Hugh Davis

AARON LEVINE: Washington, D.C., attorney who, with Bradley Post, went before the FDA's Obstetrical and Gynecological Device Classification Panel in December 1977 to ask for a recall of the Dalkon Shield

JACK LIPPES, M.D.: inventor of the Lippes Loop

MILES LORD: U.S. District judge who reprimanded three A. H. Robins executives in a Minnesota courtroom

LAZAR MARGULIES, M.D.: inventor of the Gynekoil, the first commercially sold plastic IUD

DAVID MEFFORD: quality control supervisor for A. H. Robins

KEN MOORE: project manager for the Dalkon Shield, A. H. Robins, 1971–1973

CHARLES MORTON: vice-president and general manager, A. H. Robins

GAYLORD NELSON: Democratic Senator from Wisconsin who chaired the 1970 "Pill Hearings"

BOB NICKLESS: A. H. Robins' product management coordinator, 1970; director, international marketing, 1971–1974

DONALD OSTERGARD, M.D.: California obstetrician-gynecologist who performed clinical studies on the Dalkon Shield, sponsored by A. H. Robins, to determine the Shield's pregnancy rate

FLETCHER OWEN, M.D.: director, medical services, A. H. Robins, 1970–present

ALLEN POLON: research and development program coordinator, A. H. Robins

BRADLEY POST: Wichita attorney who won the first Dalkon Shield lawsuit against A. H. Robins; lead counsel for Dalkon Shield plaintiffs' attorneys

ELLEN PRESTON, M.D.: project coordinator and physician-liaison for the Dalkon Shield, 1970–1973

LESTER PRESTON: A. H. Robins' biostatistician and director of scientific information

E. CLAIBORNE ROBINS, JR.: president and chief executive officer of A. H. Robins since 1978; board member since 1972

E. CLAIBORNE ROBINS, SR.: president and chief executive officer of A. H. Robins, 1933–1970; chairman of the board, 1970–present

JULIAN ROSS: Wayne Crowder's supervisor at Chap Stick Company

ALEXANDER SCHMIDT: commissioner of the FDA

ROY SMITH: director of product planning for A. H. Robins, 1969–1971; assistant vice-president, new product planning, 1971–1973; vice-president, new product planning, 1973–1975; senior vice-president, new product planning, 1975–present

ROBERT SNOWDEN: English sociologist who, in 1981, conducted a retrospective study for A. H. Robins on the relationship between the Dalkon Shield and pelvic infections

HOWARD TATUM, M.D.: inventor of the Copper-T who conducted experiments on the Dalkon Shield tail string in 1974, showing that it could wick bacteria into the uterus

JOHN TAYLOR: public affairs assistant, A. H. Robins, 1973–1976; director, public affairs, 1976–present

FRANK THEIS: U.S. District judge in Kansas who supervised the Dalkon Shield multi-district litigation

RUSSEL THOMSEN, M.D.: Army physician who spoke out against the Dalkon Shield at the 1973 "Fountain Hearings"; author of 1985 AID report on the agency's actions regarding the Dalkon Shield overseas

CHRISTOPHER TIETZE, M.D.: well-known contraception expert and IUD-advocate who established the life table method of evaluating IUDs

ROGER TUTTLE: A. H. Robins attorney, 1971–1976

RICHARD WILCOX: New York public relations expert who was hired by A. H. Robins to get favorable press coverage for the Dalkon Shield

LILLIAN YIN: director of the FDA's Office of Ob-Gyn Devices

WILLIAM ZIMMER: president and chief operating officer of A. H. Robins, 1970–1978

NIGHTMARE

Pam

"Because there is nothing to take, nothing to use, and nothing to remember before or after having relations, most women find the Dalkon Shield the safest and most satisfying method of contraception they have ever used. With the superior protection of this modern IUD, you can relax and enjoy the luxury of a truly superior birth control method."
> —The A. H. Robins' patient brochure for the Dalkon Shield, December 1970.

"If I had even had an inkling that I was in any danger [from the Dalkon Shield], I would never have left it in."
> —Pam Van Duyn, October 1984.

On a cool October day in 1977, 26-year-old Pam Van Duyn walked across the campus of the University of Oregon in Eugene. She stopped to rest for a moment, catching her breath, still weak from the operation she had undergone six weeks earlier.

As she watched the other students hurry past her on the way to class, she wondered how long she would feel like this. How long it would be until her strength returned and she would be able to walk the length of the campus at a brisk pace, to take a full load of classes.

She remembered her doctor's words, "Take it easy, get your strength back, just proceed one day at a time."

Taking a deep breath, Pam resumed her cross-campus trek. But after only a few steps, she began shaking uncontrollably. She remembered

1

other words from her doctor, words she had heard—and had thought she had accepted—weeks ago. But now, their impact seemed to be hitting her for the first time.

"The chances of your ever getting pregnant are very slim," her doctor had said.

Pam began to cry. She couldn't control the shaking. The fact of her infertility came crashing down on her, as if she had suddenly realized that someone close to her had died.

She ran to her car and drove to a friend's house nearby. Pam sat there for hours, crying, grieving for the children she would never have.

Pam's nightmare had started two months earlier, on a warm August night in Portland, Oregon. She and her 18-year-old sister, Jennifer, had driven up from Eugene to spend the weekend with friends. Pam's husband of four years, Jim, was in a small town 400 miles away, working on a project for the State Historic Preservation Office. He would be returning to Eugene in a few weeks, when they would both begin another year of school. Pam was finishing her undergraduate work in preparation for law school; Jim was studying architecture.

Although they were living like "starving students," Pam and Jim had a happy marriage. They both came from large families in the same small town—Baker, Oregon, where the traditional values of family life had been emphasized. They hoped to begin their own family in just a year or two, while Pam was in law school. But in the meantime, Pam wore an intrauterine device (IUD) to protect against pregnancy.

That first night in Portland, Pam went to a concert with Jennifer and their friends. When she returned to their friends' house, Pam began to feel ill. Nothing specific, just an all-around achiness. She thought it was a case of the flu coming on, so she went to bed.

Within a few hours, however, her temperature had risen to 102 degrees and her abdomen was racked with severe pain, the worst pain she had ever experienced in her life. "I literally wanted to die," Pam remembers.

The following morning, Jennifer rushed Pam to a general practitioner in Portland, the doctor of some family friends. Thinking Pam had food poisoning, he gave her a shot of penicillin and a bottle of antibiotics.

"It'll pass," he said.

That afternoon, the two sisters drove back to Pam's tiny house in Eugene, where Pam curled up in bed, waiting for the drugs to take effect. But the pain did not subside, and as the hours—and soon the day—passed, Pam began to wonder if it ever would.

2

For the next five days, she lived in agony. Her temperature rose to 104 degrees. The pain was so great she couldn't eat. She lay in the house in a semi-conscious state, praying for the drugs to start working, wondering why it was taking so long.

On Friday, the fifth day after she'd seen the doctor, Pam took the last of the pills. Early the next morning Jim called, as he had every day since she had become ill. He was already very worried, but when he spoke with Pam that Saturday morning, he realized that she was rapidly losing the ability to think clearly or make decisions.

Something was seriously wrong.

"Go to a doctor right now," he told her.

Pam and Jim had no family doctor, nor did they have any health insurance. So Pam, with Jennifer's help, searched through the Yellow Pages for a doctor. Pam specifically wanted a gynecologist this time; because of the pain's location, she suspected it might have something to do with her uterus or ovaries. Several of the doctors Jennifer called said they couldn't fit Pam in on a Saturday on such short notice.

Dr. Randall Lewis, however, agreed to see her. He was a 32-year-old obstetrician-gynecologist who had recently come to Oregon after completing his residency at the Mayo Clinic in Rochester, Minnesota. Looking back, Pam says that she couldn't have drawn a better name out of the phone book. Over the next few months Lewis would give her extraordinary care, and would bill her for only a fraction of it.

The Eugene Clinic, where Lewis worked was only a few miles away. Pam made the trip curled up in a fetal position on the passenger seat of her sister's car. Jennifer helped Pam into the doctor's waiting room and pushed three chairs together so Pam could lie down. Pam didn't wait there long. She was rushed into the doctor's examining room, where Lewis quickly gave her a pelvic exam.

Lewis recognized immediately what was wrong. It wasn't food poisoning that was ravaging Pam's body. It was an acute case of pelvic inflammatory disease (PID), an insidious disease that affects the uterus, ovaries, and other pelvic organs and, if left unchecked, can be fatal.

Lewis reached into Pam's vagina and carefully pulled on a string dangling from her cervix. A crab-shaped piece of plastic slipped out. He held it up for her to see. It was her intrauterine device—a Dalkon Shield. This was the cause of her infection, he told Pam. This was the cause of her pain.

In another two days it might also have become the cause of her death.

Lewis put Pam in the hospital immediately. Blood tests revealed that her white blood cell count was more than 15,000, indicating that her body was battling a serious infection. (The count would probably have been much higher if Pam had not been given the general antibiotics a week earlier in Portland.) X-rays revealed a large, tender mass the size of an orange attached to Pam's left ovary and Fallopian tube. This was where the ovary and tube had become stretched, distended, and matted with pus from the infection.

Pam was given a series of tests to find out exactly which organism had invaded her body. Those tests, which involved examining cultured tissue of her infected organs and of the tail string of the IUD, would take some time; for the organism would have to reproduce many times to produce a colony large enough to be examined under the microscope. In the meantime, Lewis put Pam on a broad-spectrum penicillin, hoping that it could fight off the as-yet-unknown organism.

Lewis also warned Pam that if they couldn't identify and treat the organism soon, he would have to perform a hysterectomy in order to save her life. Such an operation is a serious matter at any time, but is even more dangerous for a patient with a raging infection, such as Pam's.

Jim was called. He left for Eugene immediately, making what is normally an eight-hour drive in slightly more than six. When he reached Pam's hospital bedside, he was stunned and frightened by what he saw. "She was completely dehydrated. Her lips were parched. She had no color. She was listless," he remembers.

It was Saturday night. Surgery was scheduled for Monday. By Sunday night, the situation had not improved. The penicillin was not working. Pam's temperature remained at 102 degrees and an operation seemed inevitable.

Pam begged Lewis to do more tests, to do anything to save her from a hysterectomy. She was only 26. She and Jim wanted a family. "All I could think of was my worthlessness as a woman," she recalls.

Lewis decided to wait, partly because of Pam's pleas and partly because the Mayo Clinic had trained him to take a conservative approach to operations. He moved the surgery to Tuesday, then Wednesday. He wanted to see the results of one final culture—the one done on organic matter found on the Dalkon Shield he had removed from Pam's uterus. Those tests came back Tuesday night. Two organisms were identified: Bacteroides fragilis and peptococcus. Both are commonly found in the vagina, but not in the uterus, which has a sterile—bacteria-free—interior. Lewis suspected, however, that these two organisms were probably only accomplices to Pam's infection. The organism that had initiated the infection had most likely been eradicated by the antibiotics she had taken earlier. No matter which bacterium had initially been the culprit, Lewis

4

felt all the organisms had entered Pam's uterus by climbing up the tail string of her Dalkon Shield.

Lewis changed Pam's medication, giving her an antibiotic specifically designed to fight the bacteria in her uterus. Within 24 hours, her white blood cell count dropped to near normal. Her body was finally fighting off the terrible infection that had almost killed her.

The following Sunday, after nine days in the hospital, Pam went home. It would be three weeks before she would be strong enough to get out of a bed. She still had her uterus and ovaries and Fallopian tubes, but they had been badly damaged. Her right Fallopian tube and ovary were heavily scarred from the infection. And the orange-sized mass of distended tissue, although no longer containing pus, remained attached to her left ovary and Fallopian tube. It was like carrying a time bomb. It might heal itself, as Lewis had seen in other patients at the Mayo Clinic; or it might flare up again and send Pam back to the hospital.

As she was preparing to leave the hospital, Lewis told her that with such scarring it was unlikely that she would ever bear a child. Pam had been too ill at the time to comprehend what that meant to her. She was simply grateful that the pain had ended, that she was still alive.

It was as she walked across the University of Oregon campus six weeks later that Pam fully understood the significance of Lewis' statement that she probably never would have children. She had always been a strong woman, but now she felt out of control. She had become a victim.

What Pam didn't realize was that her suffering, both physical and mental, was just beginning. In the coming years, the company that made the device that caused her agony would attack her in court as a woman with venereal disease who hadn't really wanted to have children anyway. Her marriage, torn by her physical and mental stress, would almost be destroyed. And, as she feared, she would return to the hospital time and time again to save her health and to try to improve her slim chance of having the children she so much wanted.

The device inserted in Pam Van Duyn—the Dalkon Shield—was meant to bring women freedom from pregnancy. But for thousands of women, it instead brought a prison of pain. Like Pam, many suffered severe and debilitating side effects: bleeding, inflamed and perforated uteri, unplanned pregnancies, spontaneous abortions, and premature deliveries. Some became sterile and infertile. Others delivered babies with birth defects. At least 20 women have died.

This tragedy should never have happened. And it wouldn't have if the manufacturer of the Dalkon Shield, the A. H. Robins Company, had acted responsibly. Although A. H. Robins did not set out to market a dangerous product, the prospect of profits and a stubborn refusal to admit to anything that might tarnish its reputation blinded the company to early warnings that the device presented a serious health risk to the women who used it. At first, the company ignored these warnings; later, it chose to conceal them.

A. H. Robins, however, is not the only irresponsible player in this tragedy. During the four years the Dalkon Shield was on the market (1970–1974), relatively few physicians spoke out about the complications their patients were suffering as a result of the Shield. Yet one women's health organization estimates as many as 500,000 women may have been injured by the Dalkon Shield.

Nor did the federal government take quick and active steps to remedy the problem. The Food and Drug Administration waited four years after the first reports of trouble to take a serious look at the Shield and its problems. And after the defective device was withdrawn from the market, the FDA did nothing to see that the Shield was removed from the women already wearing it.

Lawyers, too, have often played a less-than-honorable role in this story. Eager to make a quick dollar, many have given Dalkon Shield victims assembly-line treatment. Several attorneys got into serious legal trouble for making questionable payments to an insurance adjuster with whom they were negotiating settlements of Dalkon Shield claims. Other attorneys gathered large numbers of Dalkon Shield clients through advertising and then settled the cases as quickly as possible for whatever they could get.

Attorneys working on behalf of A. H. Robins have routinely humiliated women in cross-examination, asking detailed and irrelevant questions about their sexual and personal hygiene habits. Knowing they faced such intimate questions if they challenged A. H. Robins in court, many women have chosen instead to settle for whatever compensation the company would give them.

The story of the Dalkon Shield is a story of corporate greed and blind consumer trust, of government ineffectiveness and medical apathy. Above all, however, it is the story of 2.2 million American women (approximately 3.2 worldwide) who were used as guinea pigs for a product that should never have left the laboratory—and of the thousands of women who suffered as a result.

Women like Pam Van Duyn.

2

Pebbles, Pessaries, and Population Bombs

"I have often stated to my patients that the only difference between the stone placed in the womb of the camel and the intrauterine device of today is the material, and there is no evidence that one is safer than the other."
——Dr. John G. Madry, Jr., testifying before a congressional subcommittee, May 30, 1973.

In the spring of 1962, when Pam Van Duyn was still a child attending grade school in Baker, Oregon, a small group of doctors from around the world gathered in a conference room in New York City (the conference was officially called the First International Conference on Intra-uterine Contraception) to discuss the future of intrauterine devices.

Only a few years earlier, IUDs had been a dead issue as far as most gynecologists were concerned, for the unpopular contraceptive devices had been plagued by persistent reports that they caused bleeding and dangerous infections in the women who used them.

New studies and technological advances, however, had revived interest in IUDs. Reports of hundreds of women in Europe and Israel and thousands in Japan wearing IUDs without major complications had begun to surface in 1959, causing quite a stir in the gynecological community.

Maybe the IUD had been wrongly maligned in the past. Maybe it deserved another look.

Maybe this time it would prove safe.

Advocates of the IUD had long been promoting it as the ultimate

7

contraceptive. No need to stop at a passionate moment and fumble for a condom or diaphragm. No need to worry about counting days, or taking pills, or using messy foams or gels. Once inserted in the uterus, the IUD could be forgotten. Sex could be spontaneous, and, IUD advocates contended, worry-free. And because it didn't require a woman to do anything for it to be effective (after all, a woman could not forget to use the device once it was in place), the IUD was also seen as one of the last great hopes for stemming the growing tide of humanity that threatened to overwhelm the world.

Simple. Safe. Effective. Those were the claims heard at that 1962 conference. They had, however, been heard before. Indeed, for centuries men have tried—and claimed success at—stopping conception by inserting objects into women's uteri. Legend says the idea began with Arab and Turkish camel drivers who pushed small round stones into their animals' uteri to prevent their camels from getting pregnant on long sojourns across the desert. If a camel became sick or died, it was, no doubt, considered retribution from the gods for some sin the camel driver had committed.

In pursuance of this theory of contraception, more than stones have been used in women. Early IUDs were apparently fashioned out of whatever material struck the inventor's fancy. Ebony, glass, ivory, wood, pewter, wool, and even diamond-studded platinum were stuck into the uteri of women. In the 17th century, the Italian adventurer Casanova recommended the use of a gold ball. It is not known how many women acted, at the time, on Casanova's suggestion; however, as recently as 1950 one woman successfully used her gold wedding ring as a do-it-yourself IUD for almost three years.

The true forerunner of the modern IUD was the cervico-uterine pessary, a T-shaped device often made of metal. It was a cousin of the more common vaginal pessary that had initially been designed to help a woman with a prolapsed uterus—a womb that had slipped into the vagina; or, in extreme cases, out of the body. A prolapsed uterus used to be one of the most serious medical problems experienced by women. The condition was mostly due to a combination of poor obstetric care and poor diet, although doctors often blamed it on girdles, too much sex, and such activities as singing, dancing, and horseback riding.

The standard vaginal pessary was also T-shaped and filled the vagina with its donut-shaped head pressing against the cervix to keep the uterus in place. Somewhere along the way, however, someone got the idea to turn the device around and stick the stem into the uterus. (Perhaps the idea came from reading Hippocrates. He had recommended putting two small olive-sized pessaries made of plant resin and dipped in rose or iris oil into a woman's uterus to keep it in place.) Soon it was claimed that in addition to giving the uterus support, these cervico-uterine pessaries could cure a potpourri of other female complaints, including infertility, low sex drive, painful menstruation, and "hysteria." Cervico-uterine pessaries took many shapes. Some looked like buttons, some looked like screws. One of the more dangerous versions was shaped like a wishbone with a split spring that opened up within the uterus (and often perforated it).

Although it was purported that cervico-uterine pessaries encouraged pregnancy, women soon began to realize that the devices were actually preventing conception, especially when the stem accidently broke off and remained in the uterus, as frequently happened. Some women found that the devices could be used to induce abortion and many women, desperate to end a pregnancy, used cervico-uterine pessaries for just that purpose. Soon women were having pessaries inserted for contraceptive reasons alone, although neither they nor their doctors openly admitted it. In America, dispensing contraceptive devices—or even information on the subject—was against the Comstock Law of 1873. Although the law's main intent was to keep obscene or pornographic materials from getting in the hands of the public, it also prohibited people from mailing or carrying contraceptive devices and literature across state lines. The law made it a crime to disseminate any information about birth control; it remained in effect for more than 50 years. Even medical journals were reluctant to publish articles on the subject for fear that volumes containing such articles would be seized by the government.

Several doctors were arrested under the Comstock Law for dispensing contraceptives. But while prescribing cervico-uterine pessaries for contraceptive reasons presented doctors with the risk of going to jail, women who used them were literally risking their lives. Penicillin, the first antibiotic, did not become available until 1942, and in those pre-antibiotic days any infection that developed in the uterus could quickly become disastrous. In 1924, one doctor reported 385 cases of pessary-related illnesses, including several deaths. Soon, the more responsible members of the medical profession began to view the use of cervico-uterine pessaries as dangerous quackery.

The first "modern" IUD made a brief, modest—and illegal—appearance on the medical scene in 1909. It was the brainchild of Richard Richter, a doctor who practiced in what is now the Polish village of Waldenberg near Breslau. His device consisted of two or three looped rings of silkworm gut, a material commonly used at the time to suture

9

wounds. The loops were joined together by a short piece of aluminum-bronze wire, which, with the silken ends of the loops, formed a kind of "tail." The entire device was poked into the uterus with the aid of a wooden stick. When the stick was removed, the ring would be left in place with its wire-and-silk tail dangling in the upper part of the cervix. Richter could then use the tail to pull the device out of the uterus if such a need arose.

It's not clear how many of Richter's devices had to be removed for reasons of infection or excessive bleeding. Nor is it known exactly how effective his IUD was. Many European countries had contraception laws similar to the Comstock Law, and Richter did not keep records of pregnancies or infections among his IUD users, probably because such records could have been used to put him in jail.

Richter did feel that he could write about the device safely, however, and in 1909, he proudly announced his new invention in a German medical journal. In fact, he felt compelled to write about the device, for malnutrition was common in his region and he had witnessed its dire effect on women who were forced to bear children year after year out of contraceptive ignorance. "One who knows life as it is," Richter wrote, "knows also that hundreds of mothers sacrifice their health and happiness every year for the sake of childbearing . . . It becomes a matter of obligation and conscience under these circumstances for the physician to restrain the excess of children." Richter believed his invention would provide that needed restraint. "After many years of testing and improving," he declared, "I am able to offer to my colleagues a simple and safe contraception."

Richter's invention was largely ignored by the medical community—probably because of its illegality—and not much was heard about IUDs for the next 14 years. Then, in 1923, a German doctor, Karl Pust, used three twisted strands of silkworm gut to create a new IUD. Shaped somewhat like a baby's pacifier, its tail of dangling silken strings was wrapped tightly with yet another silk thread and then attached to a button of glass. (Pust thought the glass button would aid the contraceptive effect of his device by discouraging sperm from entering the uterus.) In many ways, Pust's IUD was a kind of cross between Richter's silkworm ring and the old pessaries.

Pust claimed he had followed the history of 453 women who had his device inserted and that *not one* had become pregnant or had a serious complication. Reports from other doctors, however, soon told another, more painful, story. It seemed that the silk-wrapped tail drew bacteria from the vagina into the uterus, causing life-threatening infections. More than 20,000 of Pust's IUDs were distributed before the device was finally condemned by the medical profession. How many of those women became ill or died is not known. Several aspects of the Pust episode—the glowing initial reports from the inventor, the tail strings causing infection, the injuries to women—were hauntingly similar to events that would occur 50 years later with the Dalkon Shield.

Despite the horrific tales that pursued Pust's device, interest in IUDs did not wane, but grew. Doctors in several countries, encouraged by a growing acceptance of birth control, eagerly began to experiment with different designs. In the pre-Pill days of the '30s and '40s IUDs were seen as birth control's greatest hope. Wrote one enthusiastic inventor, "[The IUD] is free from the aesthetic disadvantages of all other methods of contraception, and does not interfere at all with the spontaneity of intercourse. It requires no preparation just before intercourse, which may take place equally well in the marital bed or on the sea-shore."

Feminists of the day also eagerly embraced the new devices, which they saw as a way of freeing women from the economic bondage of too many children. In fact it was Margaret Sanger, the leader of the growing birth control movement, who helped organize the 1930 International Birth Control Conference in Zurich at which an IUD was a star attraction.

The inventor of this new IUD was Ernst Grafenberg, a German ophthalmologist-turned-gynecologist with a practice on Berlin's fashionable Kurfurstendamm. He took Richter's concerns about the medical emancipation of women one step further and claimed IUDs would free women from sexual inhibitions as well as from the bondage of too many children. "A satisfactory contraceptive method is most important in dealing with psychosexual disturbances in women," he announced at one presentation of his IUD to colleagues. "By removing fear and the necessity for objectionable preparations, many physical and mental inhibitions are removed."

Grafenberg's device was a simple ring of "German silver," which was a mixture of copper, zinc, and silver. Unlike earlier IUDs, Grafenberg's ring had no tail string, for the doctor was convinced that tail strings were the culprits in pessary infections, providing "a path whereby germs from the vagina many enter the uterus." Grafenberg reported that he had inserted 600 of his silver rings into his patients and that less than two percent of the women had become pregnant. He did not mention infections, although a year earlier, in reporting on a smaller group of 150 insertions, he had claimed that the ring had not caused a single infection.

Grafenberg was the first IUD inventor to give full and clear instructions about how his devices were to be inserted and removed. He insisted that all equipment used to insert the IUD be sterilized to avoid introducing an infection to the uterus. He said a pain killer, or anesthetic, was unnecessary before insertion; in fact, Grafenberg thought the anesthetic would be more traumatic to the patient than the insertion. He also stressed that his ring was not suitable for all women, especially women who had a pre-existing vaginal infection, such as gonorrhea.

Grafenberg's IUD presentation was not well received in Germany, where all contraception was soon to be banned under the Nazi regime. (The Nazis, after all, wanted the Aryan race to be fruitful and multiply to take over the world, not to limit their families; official Nazi policy encouraged both married and single women to bear as many children as possible.) In 1931, Grafenberg's research was denounced by almost all of Germany's leading gynecologists and IUDs virtually disappeared from German medical practice. The Grafenberg ring, however, enjoyed a brief acceptance in other countries and soon became fashionable among women who could afford it and who were willing, in some instances, to break the law to wear it.

Fashionable perhaps, but not safe. Many women hoping to find freedom through Grafenberg's ring, instead found infection and pain. Grafenberg's thoroughness in investigating and reporting on his ring eventually brought him the title "father of the IUD"; but, unfortunately, no one else could match his clean results with the device. A Copenhagen doctor reported in 1932 that 50 of the 178 Grafenberg rings he inserted had to be removed "because of constant bleeding, pain, discharge and tenderness." Although he had begun as an enthusiastic supporter of the ring, the doctor concluded that "my experiences lead me to feel that I would not myself use the intrauterine means in public clinics, for which I prefer the perfectly harmless and very safe rubber vaginal caps." Dr. Norman Haire, a well-known London (via Australia) gynecologist, also reported problems with the ring. He had once denounced intrauterine devices but had since become a staunch supporter of Grafenberg. Of the 400 devices Haire inserted in 1931, 20 percent were expelled and 10 percent failed to keep the women who wore them from getting pregnant. In spite of these problems, Haire continued to recommend the device until 1952, when he finally conceded that its problems outweighed its benefits.

By 1937, the year Grafenberg escaped the Nazis and emigrated to New York, these and other reports of infection—and of at least one death—had made his device bitterly controversial outside as well as inside Germany. A standard textbook on contraception, published in 1938, labeled the Grafenberg ring "harmful," and strongly recommended against its use.

Upon the advice of friends who feared he would be censured by the American medical community, Grafenberg quietly withdrew himself from the IUD controversy once he arrived in the United States. Although he continued to insert IUDs into his private New York patients, he apparently refrained from using them at the Margaret Sanger Clinic, where he also saw patients. To them, his more "public" patients, he prescribed cervical caps and diaphragms until his death in 1957.

In 1936, the Comstock Law was effectively overturned by the courts, and disseminating birth-control information became legal again. Encouraged by the more liberal attitude and convinced they could overcome the infection problem, a few IUD advocates pushed on with their experiments. One such advocate was Tenrei Ota, a Japanese doctor who, like Grafenberg, began experimenting with IUDs in the 1920s. The Ota Ring, as his device became known, went through many permutations, from a solid gold ball in 1927 to a plastic spiral by the mid-1960s. The device that still bears his name is a coiled ring of either silver, gold, or plastic with two or three radial arms suspended within it. It looks somewhat like the steering wheel of a car. Ota first reported on his device in 1934, saying he had inserted it in 73 women with only one pregnancy. No mention was made of infections, and the Ota Ring soon became very popular among Japanese gynecologists.

In the Western world, however, IUD experiments went largely unheralded. Between 1934 and 1959, only one paper on IUDs appeared in English in any of the important medical journals. That paper, although favorably disposed toward IUDs, made little impression on the medical world, and they were all but forgotten by most physicians and certainly by the public.

In 1959, however, all that changed. That year, an Israeli doctor, Willi Oppenheimer, announced that he had been fitting two ring devices, including the Grafenberg ring, in several hundred private patients since 1930 with exceptionally good results. A similar report about the Ota Ring came out of Japan that same year, but in that report the number of women reportedly fitted with the IUD was in the thousands.

The medical profession was stunned. Suddenly it seemed as if the condemnation IUDs had received over the decades had been unfounded, perhaps even hysterical. Almost overnight, the idea of putting a foreign object into the sterile uterus and leaving it there became acceptable.

Two major technological advances of the 1950s helped spur this acceptance. One was the development of antibiotics. Armed with such new drugs as penicillin, tetracycline, and streptomycin, doctors lost their fear of pelvic infections. If an infection flared up in an IUD patient, a simple shot or two of an antibiotic could now take care of the infection before it spread throughout the abdomen—most of the time.

The availability and versatility of plastic was the other technological advance that caused doctors to become more open to IUDs. Plastic IUDs were inert, which meant they didn't interact chemically with the body. Once placed in the uterus they would not change into another form, give off toxins, or deteriorate—or so it was believed. Plastic IUDs were also more flexible than those made of metal. They could be given what engineers call "memory"—the ability to return to their original shape after being stretched during insertion into a woman. Doctors were tremendously impressed with this breakthrough, for it meant they would no longer need to dilate—open—a woman's cervix before inserting an IUD. With all the earlier devices, including the Grafenberg ring, doctors had had to insert a series of metal rods of increasing width in the opening of a woman's cervix to create a space wide enough for the IUD to pass through. Although Grafenberg insisted the procedure didn't require a local anesthetic, other doctors found it too painful for their patients to undergo the procedure without one. And giving any anesthetic presents some health risk to women. Some women break out in rashes or asthma symptoms as the result of being exposed to an anesthetic; in rare instances, a woman may suffer a heart attack or stroke.

Plastic made the process vastly simpler. A plastic IUD could be stretched into a long and narrow shape and then slipped through the cervix and into the uterus. Once inside, it would "spring" back into its intended shape. Fitting a patient with an IUD now became a routine procedure that could be done within minutes in a doctor's office.

Inventors—mostly doctors working independently in clinics and hospitals—went to work quickly. Plastic IUDs shaped like bows, coils, loops, butterflies, and spirals sprang to life in a quest for the "perfect" IUD. Thousands of women became unknowing or ill-informed guinea pigs for the physician-experimenters, often with painful results. Several of these devices, for example, had the nasty habit of perforating the uterus and finding their way into the intestine, where they painfully obstructed the bowel. Women would have to be strapped to an operating table to have the "lost" IUDs found and removed. Other women were to arrive in hospital emergency rooms, bleeding and doubled over in pain as their bodies tried to expel the IUDs. One doctor at New York's Mt. Sinai Hospital, where much experimenting with IUDs was conducted in the early 1960s, recalls that he first learned about IUDs in the hospital's

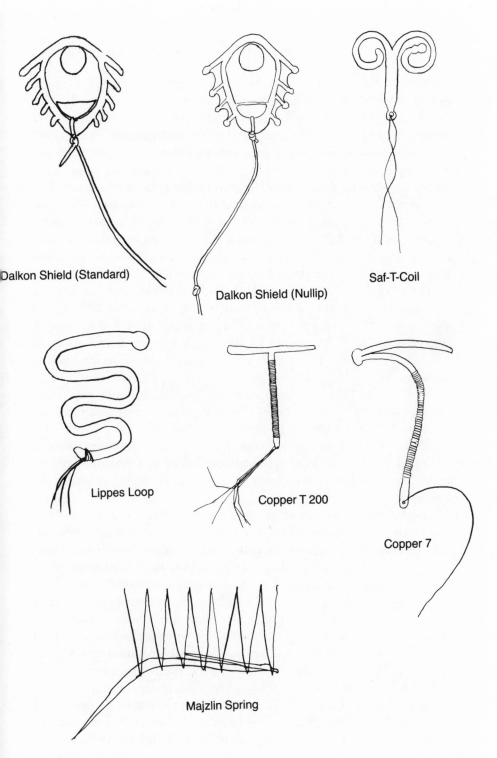

Dalkon Shield (Standard)

Dalkon Shield (Nullip)

Saf-T-Coil

Lippes Loop

Copper T 200

Copper 7

Majzlin Spring

15

emergency room, where women arrived "with strings hanging out of their cervix" and complaining of bleeding and cramps.

At the 1962 conference, however, these stories of pain went mostly untold. Instead, the doctors heard laudatory reports from such IUD inventors as New York's Dr. Lazar Margulies, who for two years had been fitting patients with a snail-shaped device that later, under the trade name Gynekoil, became the first commercially sold plastic IUD; and from Dr. Jack Lippes, a Buffalo gynecologist whose plastic loop device would soon become the standard that other IUDs would be measured against.

The 1962 conference was a turning point in IUD history—the moment, really, when the genie was let out of the bottle. It was a calculated release, engineered by the Population Council, an organization concerned, indeed obsessed, with the world's growing population. Founded in 1952 by John D. Rockefeller III and supported by the United Nations Fund for Population Activities and the Ford and Rockefeller foundations, the nonprofit Population Council believed, as Rockefeller himself had stated, that "the problem of unchecked population growth is as urgently important as any facing mankind today . . . It becomes a central task of our time to stabilize this growth soon enough to avoid its smothering consequences."

By 1962, the ticking terror of a coming "population bomb" was showing up more and more in the headlines in magazines and newspapers. Thomas Malthus' nightmarish prediction, made 160 years earlier, of a world over-peopled and underfed seemed to be coming true. Between 1930 and 1960, a billion people had been added to the world's population. Great food wars and famines were said to loom just over the horizon.

Most of the fears centered on the developing nations of Africa, Asia, and South America, but the United States was also seen as becoming too crowded. During the 1960s, the country's population exceeded 200 million—a psychological as well as a statistical milestone. Where would all these people live, work, and play? The country's—indeed the world's—population appeared galloping toward doom. By the end of the 1960s, it seemed to be on everyone's mind. Even television's Johnny Carson got in the act, holding somber midnight discussions with population expert Paul Ehrlich about the perils of an overcrowded world. Millions watched the show as Ehrlich talked about his best-selling book, *The Population Bomb*, and told of how grim life would be in an overcrowded world.

It was natural, then, that the decade of the 1960s became the decade of the IUD. And the 1962 conference was the send-off for such devices. Doctors at the conference were convinced they had finally found the perfect antidote for the "population disease" and that, as one of them put it, they would "change the history of the world" by introducing the IUD.

While the mood at the conference was optimistic, there was also a sense of urgency because of the overwhelming nature of the population problem. Warren Nelson, the chairman of the conference and medical director of the Population Council, told the 42 specially selected participants that the conference had been put together within a two month period because "we felt the subject was of sufficient importance to urge that a conference be held as soon as possible." Not a month or even a week could be wasted. The new word about IUDs—that they were safe and effective—had to be gotten out.

This zealousness resulted in a very lopsided gathering. Negative reports about IUDs were quickly brushed aside as being unfounded, unreasonable, and uninformed. The conference organizers said the goal of the meeting was "fact-finding," but as the conference proceeded it seemed clear that the participants would find only those facts that they wanted to find. The evidence against IUDs was there, but it just didn't sink in. Sweeping statements were made at the conference about the safety of IUDs, statements that today seem insensitive at best.

Take, for example, the comments made by Atsumi Ishihama and Willi Oppenheimer. These were the two doctors who had triggered the new enthusiasm about IUDs by reporting their successes with the devices in medical journals in 1959. In his prepared statement, Ishihama dismisses as "superficial" any concerns about placing a foreign substance within a living uterus. "It may be an extreme position to take," he told the gathered doctors, "but it is nevertheless correct to assert that suture threads customarily used in general operations, gold crowns on teeth, dental prostheses, artificial eyes, and contact lenses can be described as foreign bodies." But Ishihama was talking about inserting something foreign into the reproductive organs of a woman, the source of life itself. One wonders whether he would have been so cavalier about inserting a device with a long history of problems into the reproductive organs of a male.

Like many of the doctors, Ishihama also played down the pain experienced by some IUD wearers. The pain of inserting an IUD, which many women have described as excruciating—worse, even, than labor pains—he simply called "a slight disturbance."

Other doctors at the conference also dismissed the pain with a remarkable callousness. Most seemed to share Oppenheimer's view that any pain experienced by an IUD wearer was not real, but "psychologically induced." Oppenheimer went even further and declared that the increased bleeding women experienced, often for many months, after an IUD was inserted was also a product of their imaginations. "It is, in my opinion, very important to convince the patient that the method is harmless," he said. "With the amount of literature that has been written in the last 30 years condemning the method, most doctors have become biased without knowing it. They have frightened the patients to such an extent that even if the patient comes to have the ring inserted because one of her friends is very satisfied, she is subconsciously frightened, watches herself more than usual, and thus often produces bleeding, which subside immediately when she is reassured and loses her anxiety." Incredibly, Oppenheimer was saying that doctors who gave credence to the medical evidence built up against IUDs over three decades were "biased." Any complaints from women of pain and bleeding were thrown back at the women and attributed to fear or neurosis, rather than to the device.

Even more disturbing was the willingness of Oppenheimer and the other doctors to brush aside other clear warning signs about IUDs.

At the conference Oppenheimer said that he had never experienced a *single* problem as a result of the 1,500 rings he had inserted. "I have never seen any complications caused by the ring—no inflammation, no fever, no heavy bleeding, and no sterility when the patient wanted to become pregnant again," he said.

That's quite a statement. Needless to say, it made a big impression on the doctors at the conference and the hundreds of other physicians who later read about the proceedings. But a closer look at Oppenheimer's statement reveals an important qualifier—caused by the ring. For Oppenheimer did see complications in his patients. He simply did not attribute them to the ring. For example, Oppenheimer attributed infections among IUD wearers to "relapses of old inflammations, which had existed before the ring was introduced, and had not been recognized in time." He admitted that he had seen such cases in his own practice. In other words, Oppenheimer dismissed any infection that showed up in IUD wearers as a pre-existing one that he or another doctor had somehow missed. How convenient. And, as later experience would show, how tragically wrong.

In this way, doctors at the conference successfully dismissed any challenge to the safety of these devices which they thought would rescue the world. Any problems reported could be viewed, in the words of one doctor, as "a matter of coincidence more than a result of wearing the device." Such self-deception helped set the stage for what was to follow with the Dalkon Shield. The ability to ignore, explain away, and even cover-up the medical realities of IUDs would reach new heights with the inventors and manufacturer of the Dalkon Shield.

Despite all of their enthusiasm for IUDs at the 1962 conference and their absolute certainty that the devices were safe and effective, Oppenheimer, Ishihama, and the other IUD advocates didn't even know how or why these devices worked.

They knew, of course, the basics of female anatomy. There is the vagina, or vaginal cavity, a muscular tube about four to five inches long. During intercourse, it receives the erect penis; it is also the cavity into which tampons are inserted, and through which an IUD must pass to reach the uterus.

At the inner end of the vagina is the cervix, a rounded knob-like organ one to two inches in diameter. In the center of the cervix is a small hole known to doctors as the "cervical os." Sperm enters the uterus through the os, which under normal conditions is usually about the size of a match tip; menstrual blood exits through it. It is the os that has to be opened, or dilated, for an IUD to pass through. However, as Margulies and Lippes demonstrated at the conference, a four-millimeter plastic

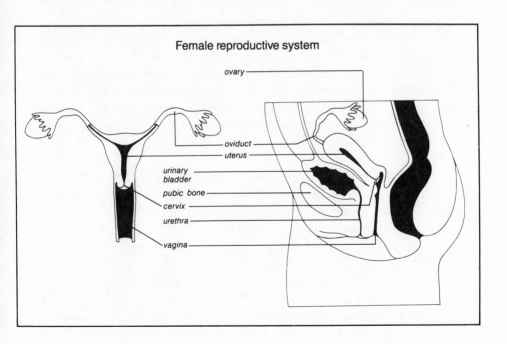

Female reproductive system

ovary

oviduct
uterus
urinary
bladder
pubic bone
cervix
urethra
vagina

straw containing an elongated plastic IUD can be poked through the os without much difficulty.

Beyond the os is the cervical canal, a short passageway that leads into the interior of the uterus. Shaped like an inverted pear, the uterus has an internal cavity that is not real space, but rather potential space. The inner walls of the uterus touch loosely, much like the pages in a book. But the walls can be pushed apart to hold an object, such as an IUD, just as a bookmarker can be slipped between the pages of a book.

Attached to the top of the uterus are the Fallopian tubes, two small, narrow tubes about five inches long and only two-tenths of an inch in diameter at their widest point. They reach out from the uterus and then curl partially back, ending in a mass of finger-like projections called fimbriae. The fimbriae, in turn, hover over the two oval-shaped ovaries that flank the uterus. Contrary to common belief, they do not "connect" the Fallopian tubes with the ovaries, for they do not actually touch the ovaries.

It is in the ovaries, of course, that human eggs are stored, some two million in all. But each month only one bursts through into the abdomen where it floats freely until it is picked up by the fimbriae and pulled into the nearby Fallopian tube. Tiny waving hair-like cells called cilia gently move the egg through the tube and toward the uterus, a journey that can take three to four days. It is in the tube that egg meets sperm and conception takes place. The fertilized egg—or burgeoning embryo—then moves on through the tube and into the uterus where it lodges in the spongy uterine wall and grows. If the egg is not fertilized, it passes out of the uterus, along with the lining of the uterus, which has been softened and laced with blood vessels in anticipation of a fertilized egg. This expulsion of the uterine lining and unfertilized egg is called menstruation.

All of this was, of course, understood at that 1962 conference. But exactly how an IUD placed in a uterus kept a fertilized egg from lodging in the uterine lining and developing was a matter of conjecture.

A quarter of a century later, scientists still can't agree on how IUDs work. Some believe the IUD irritates the uterus, making it impossible for the fertilized egg to attach itself to the lining. Others contend the irritation caused by the IUD triggers a defense mechanism that literally "eats up" either the sperm or the fertilized egg. Still others believe that the IUD mechanically loosens the egg from the uterine lining, effectively aborting it. Yet another theory is that the IUD speeds up the movement of the egg through the Fallopian tube, resulting in an egg that is too immature to successfully lodge itself in the uterine wall.

Doctors at the 1962 conference admitted their lack of understanding of how IUDs worked; but they would not admit to their lack of understanding of the connection between IUDs and pelvic infections. The prevailing belief during the 1960s—and well into the 1970s—was that IUD wearers were no more likely to develop infections of the uterus, ovaries, or Fallopian tubes than other women.

Today, there is a real concern about the connection between IUDs and pelvic inflammatory disease (PID), the modern day catch-all phrase used by doctors today to describe pelvic infections involving the uterus, ovaries, or Fallopian tubes. Studies have shown that women wearing IUDs have from 1.7 to 9.3 percent greater risk of contracting PID than non-IUD users.

Prior to widespread use of IUDs in the late 1960s and early 1970s, most PID was gonorrhea-related. With the IUD tail string providing a path for bacteria to enter the uterus, however, other, previously non-virulent, bacteria began finding their way into the sterile uterus and causing infections.

PID may come on slowly and subtly. A woman may simply feel like she is coming down with a cold or flu; with fever, chills, and a nagging discomfort in her abdomen. The symptoms may appear and disappear for many weeks or months before she realizes she has an infection. Or the symptoms may come on suddenly; with persistent and very painful cramps, high fever, nausea, fast pulse, abnormal discharge or bleeding from the vagina. If proper medical care isn't received immediately, the disease can spread into the bloodstream, causing the formation of dangerous blood clots (a condition called thrombophlebitis) or blood poisoning (a condition called sepsis). Both conditions can be fatal.

Because of the availability of medical care, death from PID is rare in the United States, but complications from the disease are not. PID can severely damage the Fallopian tubes, making it difficult or impossible for a woman to conceive. Ironically, it is the scar tissue caused by the infection, not the infection itself, that damages the Fallopian tubes. The scar tissue can either block the tubes or damage the cilia that line the inner walls of the tubes, making it impossible for the egg to travel to the uterus.

Grafenberg, of course, had warned about the dangerous connection between IUDs and PID. IUDs with tails, he noted years earlier, drew bacteria from the vagina into the uterus, with dangerous results. But IUD inventors at the 1962 conference, and later, insisted that Grafenberg was wrong. They wanted devices with tails. A tail allowed a woman and her doctor to check periodically to make sure the device was still in place, providing protection against pregnancy. It also gave a doctor something to

21

pull on, making removal of the IUD easier for the doctor, although no less painful for the patient. But, as Grafenberg had warned and the Dalkon Shield would show emphatically 10 years later, a tail could also significantly increase the danger to the women who wore the devices.

The 1962 conference was over in two brief days, but its effect on the health—or ill-health—of women was long-lasting. For it was, as one doctor later called it, "the catalyst that unleashed a burst of IUD development."

"People became convinced that the IUD was the weapon [with which] the population explosion could be dealt with," recalls Michael Burnhill, an early IUD inventor who is now professor of clinical obstetrics and gynecology at Rutgers University. "We had visions of teams of paramedics inserting these IUDs and stopping the population problem."

Burnhill admits, however, that the motives of the early IUD inventors were not totally altruistic. They were inventing these devices not only to better the social good, but to enrich themselves. "Everyone thought they were going to get five percent royalties on a million sales a year," he says.

It was not only the private consumer who would be buying these devices, but governmental agencies and private institutions, such as the Population Council, who wanted to control the world population. The market for IUDs was indeed massive. It was estimated in 1980 that as many as 60 million women worldwide were using IUDs.

IUDs cost an estimated 20 to 80 cents per device to manufacture, but are sold to private physicians for at least $15 apiece. Because groups like the Population Council now license their own IUDs, sales overseas have a much lower profit margin; but what is lost in markup is gained back, at least in part, by the vast quantities of the devices sold to developing countries.

On the optimism generated by the 1962 conference and on the promise of great profits, experiments began in earnest. Millions of women throughout the world became guinea pigs. Women from the United States were not excluded, although some doctors would have preferred to carry out the IUD tests only on the women of developing countries where malpractice laws were more lenient or non-existent.

"Experimentation with intrauterine contraceptives could be done in the countries where the legal situation is less complicated than in the United States," admitted one doctor at the conference. "However, it is completely clear that a method which is known but not used in the United States will meet very considerable resistance abroad. It will be alleged again that we, in the United States, experiment with other peoples."

Not all the women experimented on, including those in the United States, were asked to sign consent forms. Some doctors even inserted devices in women without the knowledge of the women. The doctors justified these activities to themselves and others by saying the experiments would benefit the greater good of mankind.

Whether they benefitted the greater good of womankind was—and is—another question. Perhaps the answer to that question can be found in the chilling remarks made by one of the IUD experts in the closing hour of the 1962 conference:

"We have to stop functioning like doctors, thinking about the one patient with pelvic inflammatory disease; or the one patient, who might develop this, that, or the other complication from an intrauterine device; and think of the need for this in general . . . Suppose [a woman patient] does develop an intrauterine infection and suppose she does end up with a hysterectomy and [infections]. How serious is that for that particular patient and for the population of the world in general? Not very. Perhaps we have to stop thinking in terms of individual patients and change our direction a bit . . .

. . . If we look at this from an overall, long-range view—these are things that I have never said out loud before and I don't know how it is going to sound—perhaps the individual patient is expendable in the general scheme of things, particularly if the infection she acquires is sterilizing but not lethal."

Pam Van Duyn was one of those "expendable" women. So were hundreds of young, and often poor, Baltimore women who in the late 1960s and early 1970s put their trust in a doctor named Hugh Davis.

Hugh Davis was the inventor of the Dalkon Shield.

3

The Perfect IUD

"IUDs are born in the minds of gynecologists. Be they social
humanitarians, calculating money-grabbers, or just plain
doctors hunting for the perfect mousetrap, the number of
gynecologists who have dreamed over the perfect IUD must
mount into the thousands."
                    —Russel Thomsen, M.D., testifying before a
                        congressional committee, May 30, 1973.

For Hugh Davis, the timing of the 1962 IUD conference couldn't have
been better.

The 35-year-old physician had just returned to the United States from
studying cervical cancer in Denmark and had landed an instructor's position at Baltimore's prestigious Johns Hopkins University. For Davis the
job meant returning to familiar ground; he had received his M.D. at
Johns Hopkins almost a decade earlier, in 1953, and spent the next few
years completing his residency at the school before leaving for Europe.
But now, with a new Danish wife to support, he was ready to settle in at
Johns Hopkins and carve a significant place for himself at the university's
school, one of the most competitive schools in the country.

Developing a successful IUD promised to be an ideal way to leave a
mark at John Hopkins. First of all, the chairman of the ob-gyn department at Johns Hopkins, Dr. Allan Barnes, was a true believer in the
population threat and all that it implied. In 1965, addressing a group of
doctors, he expressed the depth of his concern: "The magnitude of this
particular problem almost defies description. Within a few hundred years

24

every man, woman, and child on the face of this earth will have one square yard to occupy." Yet Barnes was not a true believer in the Pill. Like many other heads of medical departments in the early 1960s, Barnes felt the risks of birth control pills far outweighed their benefits.

The early version of the Pill, while extremely effective in preventing pregnancy, contained estrogen dosages many times stronger than those prescribed for birth control pills today. This amount of the female hormone created serious health problems for the Pill users, including an increased risk of abnormal blood clotting, heart attacks, strokes, and cancer. The first indications that the Pill had serious side effects came out of Britain in the summer of 1962. This, coincidentally, was just weeks after the Population Council's IUD conference had proclaimed IUDs the risk-free contraceptive of the future. The message to doctors seemed clear—the Pill was dangerous, the IUD safe.

Johns Hopkins took this message to heart. One doctor who was a university resident in gynecology during the 1960s cannot recall prescribing a single birth control pill during his residency. Given Barnes' attitude, it's no wonder that Johns Hopkins was receptive to IUD research and experimentation.

But it wasn't only to please his boss that Davis became deeply involved in IUDs in the early 1960s. Davis was an inventor as well as a gynecologist, a man who loved to dream up mechanical solutions for medical problems. He tinkered with a great many medical inventions besides IUDs. The Davis catheter, which Davis invented before he went to Denmark, is still used today to diagnose urethral diverticulum, an infection associated with the urethra. And his device to enable women to take their own Pap tests, although never marketed in the United States, is currently being used by women in Denmark. "He was always an inventive and original thinker, a man with a very high IQ," recalls Howard Jones, who as chairman of the gynecology department at Johns Hopkins, was Davis' former boss. "He could just pick up anything and go with it," adds Robert Israel, a former colleague who worked with Davis on early prototypes of the Dalkon Shield.

For Davis, the IUD began as an invention, a problem to be solved. And as his work toward the "perfect" IUD progressed, he undoubtedly realized that money as well as satisfaction could be found in coming up with a workable finished product.

Some of Davis' friends suggest that Davis' IUD research came out of his genuine desire to ease the threat to the world of overpopulation. But just how much of a convert Davis was to the zero population movement of the 1960s is unclear. Jones and Israel, both of whom worked almost daily with Davis during that period, cannot recall a single conversation with him about the population dilemma.

Yet Davis' own writings show a man deeply concerned with the problem. As early as 1965, in a paper presented at a May 7 Johns Hopkins conference on "Social Responsibility," he would write: "The magnitude of the problem posed by the population explosion is of such overwhelming proportions that there is virtually universal agreement on the necessity for contraception. While the planned pregnancy cannot be regarded either medically or socially as a disease, the unwanted pregnancy is certainly the world's commonest ill."

Those who most needed a cure for this ailment, Davis indicated, were the poor. But he also felt these were the people who would resist it the most. Davis complained in the 1965 paper that the poorest segments of society "aren't motivated" to use proper birth control. He then referred to the low-income women of Baltimore—the same women he would later use as test patients for the Dalkon Shield—as modern day "fellahin," a term used to describe peasants of ancient Egypt.

"While the upper socioeconomic tenth of the population can and does indulge in elaborate precoital rituals to control their fecundity," Davis wrote, "the lowest socioeconomic tenth rejects such methods. This has been true since the time of the Pharaohs. Cleopatra is said to have used a vinegar-soaked sponge in the vaginal vault as a contraceptive. The fellahin, both ancient and modern, have had little interest in chemical and mechanical contraceptives. The birth rate in the city of Baltimore in 1960 reflects this fact. There were 73 births per 1,000 white females in the highest economic class aged fifteen to forty-four, while in the lowest economic class there were 133 births. Thus, the segment of the population least able to discharge the responsibilities of parenthood was producing twice as many children per annum. The difference was nearly triple in the comparable nonwhite group."

Egotistical, cigar-chomping, a connoisseur of port wine, Hugh Davis was—is—a paradoxical man. An enigma, really. To his Johns Hopkins colleagues, he could be both charismatic and rude, friendly and sullen. Friends and foes compare him to a variety of disparate people, from comedian Groucho Marx to football coach Bear Bryant to former President Richard Nixon. "He was very outspoken and he made some very strong enemies," says Georgianna Jones, a close friend and former Johns Hopkins colleague.

By the end of the Dalkon Shield story, his friends confirm, Davis would hire a bodyguard to protect him from the mythical hit men he believed drug companies were sending after him. But that would come later, after the downfall of the Shield, after his "perfect" invention was revealed to be tragically flawed. In 1962, Davis' career still stretched out before him like a long, promising journey.

At Davis' instigation, a family planning clinic was opened at the Johns Hopkins Hospital in 1964. He was directing the hospital's outpatient activities at the time and says he saw a need for a "specialty clinic dedicated to preventive gynecology."

Although Davis also saw private patients there, the clinic drew its patients primarily from the poor, black sections of Baltimore. The clinic was touted at the time as progressive, a step forward, a way the hospital could counter its elitist reputation and reach out to the community where it was located.

But there may have been another, narrower motive for setting up the clinic. Hugh Davis had begun experimenting with IUDs in 1963. By 1964 he and Edmund Jones, an employee from the Ortho Pharmaceutical Company, had developed a newly designed IUD. They would need a place to test that device. What could be better than a specialty clinic dedicated to preventive gynecology? For at Johns Hopkins, "preventive gynecology" meant the IUD.

Although Davis has never directly said that the clinic was set up to test IUDs, he has admitted that the Ortho Pharmaceutical Company helped get the clinic started, an indication that at least one of the clinic's purposes was to provide a setting for testing the new IUD. According to Robert Israel, who was a resident physician at the Johns Hopkins Hospital at the time, the clinic's major emphasis was "to evaluate prototype IUDs."

All sorts of plastic IUDs were tested at the clinic—hard devices and soft ones, thick ones and thin ones, some with tails and some without. By 1968, the year testing began with the Dalkon Shield, 70 women were being fitted with IUDs each month at the clinic.

Israel remembers that he and Davis came up with many "wild ways" to try and check the position of IUDs in the uterus without putting tails on the devices or having to resort to X-rays. One early tailless device tested at the clinic had a magnet attached to it. "We would wave [another] magnet over the abdomen to see if the device was still there," recalls Israel.

That device, like many of the others, proved impractical. "Even if it [the magnet test] worked, you never knew if [the IUD] was in the uterus or not," explains Israel. In other words, the device could perforate the uterus and make its way into the abdomen without the doctors' being aware that it had "migrated."

In the early days of the clinic, the IUD that Davis was most interested in testing was the one he and Edmund Jones of the Ortho Pharmaceutical Company had developed—the INCON (from INtrauterine CONtraceptive). The device went through a variety of shapes as it was developed—at one point it was even tailless—but its shape in May 1966, when a patent was finally applied for it, was that of a heart-shaped shield, open, without a central membrane. The INCON was even nicknamed by Davis the "B shield" and the "heart shield."

Although the INCON was extensively tested at Johns Hopkins and a patent was finally obtained for it in 1969, it was never put on the market. It's not clear exactly why not, although the INCON had a high expulsion rate—16 percent. The device's open loop design may have also had something to do with it. By the late 1960s, open IUDs were viewed with suspicion by the medical profession. If these devices perforated the uterus, as they sometimes did, and made their way into the abdomen, they could wrap themselves around folds in the intestine and "strangle" it, much as a rubber band would. Emergency surgery would then be required to remove the device and stop the life-threatening blockage to the intestine. Whatever the reasons, by the fall of 1967 it became clear that the INCON device was going nowhere, and Davis was notified that his clinic was about to lose its funding from the Ortho Pharmaceutical Company to research and develop a new IUD.

Many men might have given up. But Davis had an idea, and he had somewhere else to turn for funding and help—his friend and fellow inventor, Irwin "Win" Lerner.

It was through his other medical inventions, not his IUD work, that Davis had first met Win Lerner, a Connecticut electrical engineer and a self-styled inventor. Davis met Lerner in the early 1960s while Lerner was working for Clay Adams, a New Jersey hospital supply and equipment company. Lerner contacted Davis and said he was interested in Davis' home Pap smear test. The American Cancer Society was testing the device and Lerner thought Clay Adams should buy and market it. The company decided against the purchase (apparently because the device could not get FDA approval), but Davis and Lerner hit it off and the promise of a partnership was born.

It was a perfect match. Davis was a doctor with a mind full of inventive mechanical ideas for the medical field. Lerner had the technical know-how to get them out of the idea stage and into production.

Within months of their meeting, Lerner quit his job at Clay Adams. He says he had no immediate plans, but was toying with the idea of starting a business of his own. The medical supplies field was wide open at the time, with big opportunities for growth. The 40-year-old Lerner wanted to jump into the field while the growth potential remained large and while he was still a relatively young man.

But where to begin? What product could he sell?

As chance would have it, Hugh Davis dropped by Lerner's Connecticut home a week after Lerner left Clay Adams. Davis told Lerner about an invention he had been working on for several years, one that would be perfect to get Lerner's new company off the ground. It was a cytology fixative, an aerosol spray that preserves a Pap smear until it reaches a laboratory. Lerner accompanied Davis back to Baltimore, took a look at the fixative, and liked what he saw. Within weeks Lerner Laboratories was founded with the fixative as its first product. The product was a hit, and in 1964 Lerner Laboratories was off and running.

During the next four years, Lerner developed many other products for his company, including several with the aid of Hugh Davis. These products included a table model centrifuge that separates the various parts of blood cells; a glue-like mounting medium that helps affix a cover glass to a microscope slide containing a biological specimen; and a cytology scraper for Pap smears. Davis received a royalty for his work on the original cytology fixative. For his consulting work on the other products, Lerner says Davis was given stock in Lerner Laboratories.

When the Dalkon Shield rolled around, however, the financial relationship between Lerner and Davis changed dramatically.

Both Davis and Lerner say they first discussed the idea for developing a new shield-shaped contraceptive during the 1967 Christmas holidays. Their families had begun a tradition of spending the holidays together, and that year they gathered at Lerner's Connecticut home.

Lerner recalls that Davis was frustrated about his IUD work. Every time he made an advance in the design of an IUD, Davis told Lerner that Christmas, someone else would come out with an advance as good and he would have to go back and try and make his even better. Only now, with his funding cut off, he wouldn't have the chance to try again. Davis suggested that Lerner, through Lerner Laboratories, attempt to design a new and improved IUD. Lerner was intrigued. It sounded like a project he and his company could get behind.

It also sounded like a project that could make a sizeable amount of money. Within weeks, Davis and Lerner drew up an agreement providing that if Lerner successfully developed and marketed an IUD, Davis would receive five percent of all net sales of the device for his help in developing and testing the device. Despite their work together on other projects, it was the first time they had set up such an arrangement.

Lerner went to work immediately on designing an IUD. He insists that he started from scratch with his design, that he did not simply modify the INCON. Davis, too, argues that the two devices had nothing to do with each other. Yet the INCON looked remarkably like the Dalkon Shield, the device that Lerner was soon to come up with. It appears, at least in basic shape, to be the skeleton upon which the Dalkon Shield was built.

Would it have made any difference if the INCON was an early prototype of the Shield? It might have made a difference to Johns Hopkins and the Ortho Pharmaceutical Company—and to the pocketbooks of Davis and Lerner. For Johns Hopkins and the Ortho Pharmaceutical Company owned the patent to the INCON; it had been assigned to them by Davis and his former partner, Edmund Jones. So, had Davis and Lerner acknowledged that their new device was simply a modified version of the INCON, they might have had a patent fight on their hands.

During the first half of 1968, Lerner labored hard to come up with a workable IUD. He had no training in gynecology and except for some earlier work on a catheter, had never before designed a product meant to be inserted into the human body. The material Lerner eventually settled on for the Shield was ethylene vinyl acetate copolymer, or EVA. It was chosen because it molded easily, was porous, inert, strong, and available in various formations so a manufacturer could select the exact amount of hardness or flexibility that was wanted.

While Lerner believed the plastic had the added benefit of being nontoxic, no one had actually tested the material for toxicity. EVA had been approved by the FDA for use in packaging materials for food, especially meat. It had never, however, been tested or approved for insertion into the human body.

The selection of the type of plastic was tied closely to the device's design. To the basic shield shape of the INCON, Lerner and Davis added a central membrane to "close" the device and thus avoid the intestinal strangulations that had been associated with the INCON and other open devices. The membrane also gave the device broader surface contact with the inner walls of the uterus, something Davis believed would increase the device's effectiveness as a contraceptive.

Fins were put along the outside edges of the membrane to help anchor the device within the uterus. Expulsion of IUDs by the uterus was still a major problem for IUD developers—as Davis knew only too well from the failure of the INCON to stay in place within many women's wombs. But the fins on this new device worked too well. They made it more difficult for the body to expel the IUD, but they also made it more difficult for a doctor to remove the device. It was like tugging on a fish hook that had gotten caught on an underwater log.

Just as a fishing line sometimes snaps when snagged, so did the first string that Lerner put on the new IUD. These were monofilament strings, or strings made out of a single untwisted strand of plastic. The monofilament string was state-of-the-art for IUD tails at the time. It was believed that they carried little, if any, risk of "wicking" bacteria from the vagina into the uterus—Grafenberg's old concern and still a major obstacle to developing the "perfect" IUD.

But Lerner and Davis found that the monofilament string was not strong enough to withstand tugs made on it by a doctor during removal of their finned device. So they tried to come up with a new improved string—a multifilament string comprised of 200 to 400 strands surrounded by an open-ended plastic sheath.

The multifilament string itself was much stronger than a monofilament string, and it did not break off during removal. However, Lerner and Davis thought that it might be more inclined to harbor potentially dangerous bacteria in the spaces between its filaments—bacteria that might then be drawn, or wicked, into the sterile uterus. They hoped the sheath would prevent this problem.

Davis was particularly concerned with the problem of wicking, for he specifically instructed Lerner to find a string that would not wick. Lerner looked at a variety of materials, finally settling on one known as Supramid, a suture material covered with translucent nylon. It was manufactured in Germany, where it was primarily used to repair tendons in horses.

Lerner tested the Supramid string for wicking. First he tied a knot about one centimeter from the bottom of an eight-centimeter-long piece of string. Such a knot would be needed on the finished model of the IUD to help doctors know that the device hadn't slipped from its preferred position high in the uterus. Lerner then dipped the lower end of the string into a test tube containing ink-dyed water. If the string wicked, it would be easy to see as the dyed water rose up the string. The multifilament Supramid string did wick. Lerner says the inky water reached the first knot. But it didn't go any further, at least in these tests, and that was apparently enough assurance for Lerner and Davis. They decided to use the string.

Never during the entire life of the Dalkon Shield, from the time it was first put in women in 1968 until it was removed from the market in 1974, did Lerner, Davis, the A. H. Robins Company, or the FDA conduct a wicking study using bacteria rather than ink-dyed water. It would take a skeptical outsider—a scientist from the Population Council—to initiate such a test in 1974. The only wicking study other than Lerner's conducted while the Dalkon Shield was being inserted in women was done by an A. H. Robins lab technician who found that there was indeed a problem. He issued warnings to A. H. Robins officials, but they were not heeded.

After deciding on the Shield's material, shape, and string, Lerner took a look at how the device could be inserted into the uterus. He experimented with the "soda straw" technique used by Jack Lippes and other recent IUD inventors for their devices. But the flat, solid shape of the Shield did not lend itself to being drawn into a "straw" and then released with a plunger-like action.

For the Shield, Lerner was forced to return to Ernst Grafenberg's old inserting method—a rigid inserter stick. He updated the method, however, by using rigid plastic rather than steel. The Shield was hooked onto the inserter stick at one end so both stick and Shield could be pushed simultaneously through the vagina and cervical os and on into the uterus. Once the Shield was in the uterus, a doctor need only rotate the stick for the Shield to become unhooked, and then remove the stick.

Lerner believed the stick inserter offered doctors more control over placement of the IUD in the uterus than the soda straw inserter. The stick resembled a uterine sound—a device used to measure the depth of the uterus—and thus would be more familiar to doctors. Lerner was not concerned, as others later were, about the stick's protruding tip. For the Shield was not attached to the stick at its end, but rather, about a quarter-of-an-inch down from the end. In their eagerness to insert the Shield high in the uterus, doctors would later find it all too easy to poke through the uterine wall with that protruding tip.

By the end of the summer of 1968, both Lerner and Davis felt they had come up with a "final" version of their IUD. Although Davis had been testing early versions on his patients at his family planning clinic, a full-fledged study was now needed.

Lerner had several hundred Dalkon Shields molded at the Pee Wee Plastic Company in Brooklyn, New York. With these Shields, Davis began in September a 12-month medical study that was to become the key piece of promotional material used to convince doctors that the Dalkon Shield was indeed the "perfect" contraceptive. Davis was able to conduct this study as part of the clinic's ongoing evaluation of contraceptives.

It was this study—later revealed to be both inaccurate and deceptive—that led to widespread acceptance and use of the Shield by physicians throughout the country.

There are strong indications that the method of selecting the women in the study was haphazard at best. Davis presented the study as being "prospective"—that is, he claimed women were chosen for the study at the time they had their Dalkon Shields inserted, before it could possibly be known how their bodies would react to the devices. But much later he admitted that some women were added to the study after the outcome of their experiences with the IUD was already known to him. This would make the study partly "retrospective"—and questionable to many researchers. For Davis could have decided to include only those women whose experiences with the Dalkon Shield would make the device look good, excluding from the study those who had problems.

The study also used what is known as a "life table" method of compiling statistics. Without careful reading, this method made it appear as if the women had worn the device for a much longer period than they actually did. Although the study ran for a year, the average period of testing for each woman was only 5.5 months, a questionable amount of time for getting reliable pregnancy rate figures.

But that wasn't the only problem with Davis' scientific methods. Many of the women included in the study claimed that they were instructed by Davis to use spermicidal foam during the 10th to 17th days of their menstrual cycle; the time when women are most likely to ovulate and, thus, get pregnant. This advice certainly muddies the study's findings regarding the Shield's contraceptive effectiveness. For how could Davis know if it was the Shield or the foam that kept the women from getting pregnant?

One month after Davis began his study, Lerner applied for a patent for the Dalkon Shield, but in his name only. Hugh Davis' name was conspicuously absent from the patent application. Yet, the IUD had been his idea in the first place and he had worked closely with Lerner on design changes.

Why the omission? Lerner and Davis insist the reason was simply one of acknowledging the true inventor of the device—Win Lerner. But there may have been another reason. For decades, Johns Hopkins had considered it "undesirable" to own patents. Its patent policy, put in writing in 1948, generally gave its employees full rights to any products developed by them at the university. By late 1967, however, the university was having a change of heart and was discussing a new patent policy to be issued in February 1968. This new policy would require employees to assign to Johns Hopkins the patent on any product they invented using university "facilities, materials, equipment, staff, or time."

Davis, of course, was using all of these at the university's COFLAC

(Community-Oriented Family Life Action Center) clinic to test the new IUD he and Lerner were working on. He may have deduced that under Johns Hopkins' soon-to-be-issued patent policy he would have to turn over his royalties from the IUD to the university. Just a year earlier, in 1967, he turned over the patent for the INCON device even though the university didn't require it.

What better way to get around the Dalkon Shield's potential patent problem than to have a close friend apply for the patent and then make some other arrangement to compensate for not sharing co-ownership of the patent? That other arrangement was made in January 1969. That month, Lerner created the Dalkon Corporation. Three people received an interest in the corporation: Lerner (55 percent), Lerner's friend and attorney, Robert Cohn of Hartford, Connecticut (10 percent), and Hugh Davis (35 percent). Davis also insisted that, in the event of Lerner's death, he be given the first right to purchase enough of Lerner's stock to own at least 50 percent of the Dalkon Corporation.

Davis' 35 percent share in the new company was a lot more than the five percent originally agreed upon a year earlier. It seems reasonable to infer that this new contract was a way of giving Davis his due as co-inventor of the IUD, but in a way that got around the troubling problem of Johns Hopkins patent policy. Lerner and Davis, however, deny this. They say Lerner's name is on the patent because Lerner was the sole inventor.

The source of the name "Dalkon" remains a mystery. Lerner and Davis have never really been clear about where the name came from, but insist that it has nothing to do with the names of the Dalkon Corporation's three partners—"Da" for Davis, "l" for Lerner, and "kon" for Cohn. Davis says his only contribution to the name was his suggestion to Lerner that the syllable "con" be included to represent "contraception." Davis also says he vetoed Lerner's first choice of a name because it had involved the syllable "mal," which Davis knew carries connotations of illness and evil in Spanish, a language he speaks fluently.

In September 1969, Davis ended his 12-month study on the IUD, which he and Lerner were now calling the Dalkon Shield. The following month, Davis submitted for publication a paper on his study to the influential *American Journal of Obstetrics & Gynecology*. It was a short paper, taking up only two pages in the journal, but it made its point in glowing terms—the Dalkon Shield was "a superior modern con-traceptive."

"For the past 7 years, trials of intrauterine devices in more than 5,000 women have been under way at our institution," Davis wrote. "Constant improvements have been noted, leading to the development of modern devices of superior performance. Recent experience with a shield design approaches the ideal of combining very low pregnancy rates with minimal side effects. These modern devices are demonstrating such excellence as to justify a revision of current attitudes toward the efficacy of intrauterine devices."

The Dalkon Shield was referred to five times, including in the title of the article, as a "superior" contraceptive. Superior to the Pill. Superior to all other IUDs.

Certainly the figures Davis reported in the paper bore out this claim. Of the 640 women in whom he inserted the Shield, reported Davis, there were "5 pregnancies, 10 expulsions, 9 removals for medical reasons, and 3 removals for personal reasons." These results translated into the following statistics: expulsion rate, 2.3 percent; continuation rate, 94 percent; medical removals, 2 percent; pregnancy rate, 1.1 percent. This meant the Shield had a pregnancy rate of 1.1 percent, equal to that of most forms of the Pill and well above that for competitive IUDs. The Lippes Loop was reporting a 2.7 percent pregnancy rate at the time; the Saf-T-Coil, a 2.8 percent rate.

Davis' article was published in the "Current Investigation" section of the *American Journal of Obstetrics & Gynecology* at a time when the magazine was changing its policy as to the method of checking articles for accuracy prior to publication. During 1969 and 1970, the journal was in the process of tightening up what had been a loose policy of checking articles only when specific questions were raised by an editor. But the new procedure, which required strict "peer review" of every article to be published, was not solidly in place when Davis submitted his study in late 1969.

Davis' study slipped through the system unchecked. No physician appears to have examined the validity of his study before it was published, and few seemed to have questioned it afterward. Nowhere in the article does Davis identify himself as co-inventor of the Shield. Nor is his financial interest in the device revealed. Nor does he state that he told some of the women to use an additional form of contraception during the period when they were most likely to become pregnant. The article is presented as the work of an unbiased, scientific observer.

Davis submitted his draft of the article to the journal in October, only days after the study was completed. This meant that women who might have become pregnant in the last weeks of the study without knowing it yet, would not be reflected in his pregnancy statistics. In fact, this is exactly what happened. While the journal was considering Davis' paper,

Davis was extending the study to 14 months. A significant number of pregnancies appeared, making the actual pregnancy rate for the device at the end of the 14 months higher—more than three percent when calculated using a simple raw calculation of the data, and more than five percent when calculated using the life table method that Davis had employed. This showed the Dalkon Shield to be decidedly inferior to both the Pill and other IUDs on the market.

Davis did not, however, correct his article. He chose, instead, to stick by his final statement in the article: "Taken altogether, the superior performance of the shield intrauterine device makes this technique a first choice method of conception control."

The article was published in February 1970, at a time when doctors were intensifying their search for an alternative to the Pill. For three weeks earlier, in highly publicized congressional hearings, medical experts had resoundingly labeled the Pill as dangerous.

Ironically, the lead-off witness in those hearings was none other than Dr. Hugh Davis. His dramatic condemnation of the Pill played a crucial role in creating the "Pill scare" that swept the country after the hearings.

It was his device that benefitted most from that scare, for within a year the Dalkon Shield would become the most popular IUD on the market.

4

Linda

"If I could get my hands on Dr. Davis, I would wring his neck."

—Linda Towle

*L*inda Towle sat in the waiting room at Johns Hopkins University Hospital's family planning clinic on a warm summer's day in 1970, waiting for her best friend, Gail Bennett. The two young women had flipped a coin a few days earlier to see who would be the first to have an IUD inserted. Gail had won the toss and she was now up on the table in the doctor's examining room, having the device inserted into her uterus.

Linda wondered how the exam was going. She wished it would be over soon, for she felt uncomfortable sitting in the clinic's waiting room. A 20-year-old secretary at a Baltimore life insurance company, Linda didn't feel she had much in common with the other women sitting around her in the waiting room, most of whom were poor and black. They must be the clinic's public patients, Linda thought. Gail, on the other hand, was here as a private patient of the clinic's director, Dr. Hugh Davis.

Gail finally stepped into the waiting room. But she looked much different than she had a few minutes earlier. She was pale and crying, her face contorted with pain.

"It hurts like hell," she told Linda.

"What did the doctor say?" Linda asked.

"He said the pain will go away. Come on, I want to go home."

Linda helped Gail to the parking lot. Gail continued to cry; at times the pain was so severe that she had to stop walking. Then she began to vomit. When they reached the car, Gail sat down on a nearby curb while Linda went to unlock the passenger door.

"I'm going to faint," Gail said.

Almost immediately, her eyes rolled back and she collapsed onto the ground. Linda ran to her. Blood was seeping through her friend's white suit. Linda shouted for help and a parking attendant ran toward her.

"Get some water," Linda cried. Gail slowly regained consciousness and, when the attendant returned with the water, she took a few sips.

"I'm taking you back to the hospital," Linda said. With the attendant's help, she got Gail into the car. She drove the car right up to the hospital's door, parking it illegally as she helped Gail, still doubled over with pain, into the building.

Linda took Gail first to the emergency room, but they were sent back to the clinic to see Dr. Davis. At the clinic, Davis gave Gail a tranquilizer and a pill to lessen the pain and told her to lie down for a while to let the drugs take effect. Then he sent her home.

"Don't worry," he assured Gail, "the pain will disappear within a few days."

Gail cried all the way home.

Later that night, Linda wondered if she should go ahead and have an IUD inserted, if she wanted to subject herself to the pain and trauma Gail had gone through. Gail's experience scared her, but she was even more scared about getting pregnant. Linda had been married less than a year and things weren't going all that well. A baby at this point could really complicate things. She could go on the Pill, but she had read all those terrible things about heart attacks and cancer.

Linda decided to go ahead and make an appointment with Davis. After all, she saw herself as a strong person, both mentally and physically, better able to handle pain than her friend Gail. Her menstrual periods had always been easy and regular. She had never had any health problems. Maybe the IUD wouldn't hurt her as it had Gail.

Maybe with her, things would be different.

Linda arrived at Davis' office to have her IUD inserted a few weeks later. Gail was with her. Gail's IUD continued to give her problems—excruciating pain during her period and almost continual bleeding. She was already thinking of having it removed, and in fact would do so in a few weeks.

But both Linda and Gail were confident that things would be different with Linda. As Gail had said, "It didn't work for me, but it might for you."

Linda was led into Davis' examining room, and Gail went with her. Linda wanted her there for emotional support during the insertion.

Linda had already undressed, climbed onto the examining table and put her feet in the stirrups when Davis walked in. His manner was very impersonal and business-like. He told Linda what he had told Gail during her exam—that the IUD was a new method of birth control that was fine for young women and actually safer than the Pill. She might feel a slight pinching sensation during the insertion, he added, but she shouldn't worry about it. Then he held up the device he was going to put into her body. It looks like the jaws of an alligator, Linda told herself.

Linda had prepared herself for the insertion, but she hadn't prepared herself for an audience. Just before putting the device in—and without asking her permission or saying a word to her—Davis turned and opened the door to the examining room. Six people walked in and looked at Linda spread on the table. Linda didn't have any idea who these people were, and Davis didn't bother to tell her. She was too frightened to ask. She assumed they were doctors or nurses; during the rest of the exam Davis talked to them—and to them only—about the procedure. He said nothing more to her. Not even when she cried out in pain as he pushed the IUD through her cervix.

Linda squeezed Gail's hand hard. "Don't worry babe, it'll be over in a minute," Gail told her. Linda began to cry. The pain was awful. It felt like a pitchfork was being thrusted into her body. And there were all these strange people standing in the room, staring into her vagina.

She wanted to go home. She wanted desperately to get out of that room and go home.

"I was just a piece of meat laying on the table," Linda recalled later. "If I live to be 100, I won't forget that."

Linda bled heavily for a week. Finally, the bleeding and the cramping pain subsided. But only briefly. A month later, during her next period, the pain returned—with a vengeance.

Linda phoned Davis. He assured her that everything was all right, that the pain wouldn't last more than another period. He told her to take some aspirin. But the pain did last, hitting her hard during her next period and then again during the following period. Linda called Davis again and got him to agree to see her at his office. When she got there, Davis examined her and insisted that nothing was wrong.

Still, the pain and heavy bleeding returned each month and seemed to get worse, not better. It reached the point where Linda could barely function during her period. She wouldn't eat, sleep, or work. She lost 25 pounds, and the heavy blood loss was making her anemic.

The pain also took its toll on her marriage. When introducing her to co-workers at his office one day, Linda's husband commented that Linda "used to be a gorgeous girl until she got sick." But it was more than her appearance that had suffered. The constant pain and bleeding had made her grumpy and moody—and disinterested in sex. The problems she and her husband had experienced earlier in their marriage became more pronounced. But now Linda felt too ill to do much about it.

In July 1971, almost a year after her Dalkon Shield had been inserted, Linda went to visit her parents at their summer home on the Magothy River near Annapolis. She took long walks along the riverbank; the sun and warm air seemed to rejuvenate her.

Then her period came, and the monthly nightmare began all over again. This time Linda's mother was there to see her daughter's suffering. It frightened her. Linda lay in bed all day, curled up in terrible pain. Late one afternoon, Linda's mother decided she couldn't stand idly by and watch her daughter suffer anymore. She went next door and described her daughter's symptoms to an old family friend who happened to be a gynecologist. He came over immediately, took one look at Linda, and told her to be in his office the next morning. The Dalkon Shield would have to come out, he said. It was creating an infection.

Linda was embarrassed to be examined by a family friend, but the following morning she went to the doctor's office. The doctor warned Linda that he might have to put her in the hospital and surgically remove the IUD if he couldn't get it out in his office. Fortunately, he was able to pull the Shield out, although he cursed the whole time.

"Putting a goddamn IUD in a young girl," he muttered.

Getting the device out was excruciatingly painful to Linda, but she refused to scream. She was afraid if she made any sound, the doctor would send her to the hospital.

After the IUD was out, Linda felt weak, as if she had been kicked by a horse. A nurse gave her ice water and applied cold wet cloths to her face. The doctor prescribed antibiotics.

The removal had taken less than an hour. By the next day, despite the painful removal, she felt fine.

Linda began using a diaphragm for contraceptive protection, and she never went back to Davis. She tried to put the entire episode behind her.

In 1975, after five years of good health, Linda came down with severe stomach pains. She thought it was appendicitis so she went to the emergency room of a Baltimore hospital, where she promptly fainted. She was kept there overnight; the doctors thought she had gastritis.

Linda returned home the next day, but it would be several years before she would feel completely well again. She began to run a steady fever and experienced recurring abdominal pain. She felt ill so often that she learned how to ignore it. She had always taken pride in her physical strength; she didn't want to be looked upon as a chronic invalid now.

Linda's marriage had ended, but in 1977 she wedded a warm and gregarious businessman named Joe. They moved to Livingston, New Jersey, to start a new life together. Joe had two children from a previous marriage and Linda was helping him raise them. But she wanted a baby of her own. She threw away her diaphragm.

A few months later, while sightseeing in New York City with her husband and stepchildren, Linda had another severe attack of abdominal pain. Her temperature rose dramatically. Joe quickly drove her back to Livingston. Although it was a simmering summer day, Linda insisted upon turning on the car's heater to ward off the chills from her fever.

Joe took Linda directly to a hospital in Livingston, where doctors quickly rushed her into the operating room for emergency exploratory surgery. The surgeon found adhesions—bands of scar tissue—all over her uterus. The diagnosis was endometritis, or pelvic inflammatory disease (PID).

Frightened, Linda called up the doctor who had taken out her IUD. He reassured her that she would be all right, but once again cursed the IUD that Davis had inserted in her years before. It had undoubtedly started a chronic low-grade infection that had, in turn, caused the adhesions, he told her.

For the first time, Linda began to worry about her ability to get pregnant. She went to a fertility specialist in Livingston, and then to a second one in Baltimore when she and Joe moved back to that city in 1978. Her fears were justified. She was told that pregnancy was unlikely, maybe even impossible.

During the next four years, Linda underwent eight more operations, including hydrotubation microsurgery, an eight-hour procedure that reconstructed her Fallopian tubes. For two weeks after the operation, doctors forced a special liquid through Linda's Fallopian tubes every other day to keep them clear. It was terribly painful.

Doctors retained little hope, however, that Linda could ever get pregnant. The scarring seemed too massive. She was told to think about adoption and to give up her dream of bearing her own child. In a way, Linda was relieved to hear this. At least the struggle to get pregnant was over now; she could pick up the pieces and go on with her life.

Yet she could not let go of the frustration and sadness she felt over not being able to have a child. She became jealous of other women with young children and began to criticize them in her mind for not properly caring for them. "If that was my child," she would tell herself whenever she saw a poorly dressed child, "I wouldn't let him go out dressed like that."

Linda tried to go on with her life, to put the bitterness and frustration behind her. But increasingly her thoughts went back to the day she had the Dalkon Shield inserted—and to Davis. She felt a need to confront him, to tell him how he had ruined her life. She devised a plan. She would make an appointment with him, then when he came into the examining room she could look him directly in the eye and ask him why he had done this to her. She even envisioned herself slapping him across the face.

Linda called to make the appointment. But when the nurse asked her why she wanted to see Dr. Davis, Linda's resolve dissipated and her anger rushed out.

"When I was a very young girl," she told the nurse, "I went to Dr. Davis and I had faith in him and trusted him. Yet he put an IUD in me and I can't have a baby."

There was a pause on the other end.

"I'm sorry," the nurse said with genuine sympathy. "I'm really very sorry."

Linda hung up the phone. That was all she wanted to hear—someone saying "I'm sorry."

5

Better than the Pill

"P.S.—The complications of the Dalkon Shield (and other IUDs) make the birth control pill seem like candy. Thought you'd like to know."
—Russel Thomsen, M.D., in a letter to a
Food and Drug Administration official, January 8, 1973.

By the end of January 1970, the "Pill scare" was reaching its peak. Numerous reports and statements about birth control pills had appeared in both the scientific and popular press, sending conflicting and often frightening messages to the 8.5 million American women (and 10 million women in other countries) who were then taking the Pill.

A British study reported that one in every 2,000 women on the Pill suffered blood clots serious enough to require hospitalization. Many became permanently disabled. This study echoed an earlier FDA report that declared "a definite association" between use of the Pill and blood clotting diseases.

These negative reports were widely reported in the press. But at the same time, many popular magazines were printing pro-Pill articles. "The pill is virtually 100 percent effective," said *Bride's* magazine in December 1969. "[It] is probably the most thoroughly tested drug ever approved for use in the country."

Women were being presented with completely contradictory information on a subject that was crucial to them. It seemed impossible to make an informed decision. To clear up this confusion, Wisconsin Senator Gaylord Nelson, chairman of the Subcommittee on Monopoly of the

Select Committee of Small Business, called for hearings on the alleged dangers of the Pill. The official purpose for the hearings, which began on January 14, 1970 and continued for five days, was to look into the "present status of competition in the pharmaceutical industry." But it was the Pill that was on trial. That's what the witnesses came to talk about, and that's what the press was there to write about.

And no one made more news during those hearings than the lead-off witness, Dr. Hugh Davis.

Actually, Davis hadn't originally been on the witness list. Georgianna Jones, his colleague at Johns Hopkins and a critic of the Pill, says the committee had asked her to testify, but she didn't feel she could handle the ordeal of testifying before Congress and recommended that Davis take her place. Davis, however, was eager to jump into the spotlight. He left no doubt in the Senators' minds as to where he stood on the issue. In no uncertain terms, he condemned researchers, doctors, drug companies, and nearly everyone else who supported use of the Pill.

"I think it can be said fairly," he told the committee, "that the widespread use of oral contraceptives [that] has developed in the United States in the past 10 years, has given rise to health hazards on a scale previously unknown to medicine."

But Davis went further than simply condemning the Pill for causing fatal blood clots. He condemned drug companies and physicians for what he felt to be unwise distribution of a birth control device before it was thoroughly researched and tested. "Shall we have millions of women on the Pill for 20 years and then discover it was all a great mistake?" he asked. (Only a few years later, another physician would sit before a congressional committee and ask essentially the same question about the Dalkon Shield.)

In his testimony, Davis also implied that drug companies had been negligent in keeping women and physicians in the dark about the dangers of the Pill: "I think that there has been a good deal of delinquency in some of the mass programs in dispensing and instructing and informing people on a mass basis without warning them about the significance of leg cramps, headaches, or other warning signs that might indicate potential hazards . . . In many clinics, the Pill has been served up as if it were no more hazardous than chewing gum. The colorful brochures, movies, and pamphlets which are used to instruct women about the Pill say next to nothing about possible serious complications."

As for doctors: "These people are busy. They read the brochures and information that the drug house tends to pump into them, I am sorry to say, but that is the reality of the situation, and many of the physicians

44

practicing in good conscience and in good faith are not fully informed about some of these rather complex questions."

These comments are particularly interesting when one considers what was to happen later with the Dalkon Shield. But Davis did not merely condemn the Pill and its advocates. Throughout his testimony he promoted what he termed a "safer alternative" to the Pill—the IUD. In fact, Davis claimed the IUD was 15 times safer than the Pill.

"Some modern intrauterine devices provide a 99-percent protection against pregnancy and can be successfully worn by 94 percent of women," Davis stated. Although he did not mention the Dalkon Shield specifically by name, Davis let it be known that Johns Hopkins had been using a device for 18 months that "has proven quite effective."

He went even further. He said this new device was effective for women who had never had a child as well as for those who had. It was a major statement. Up until these hearings, IUDs had been viewed by most physicians, and certainly by the public, as not being at all suitable for younger, childless women. Their smaller uteri had trouble retaining the devices.

Davis' testimony (and his paper which would appear three weeks later in the *American Journal of Obstetrics & Gynecology*) challenged that long-held view. "Smaller devices have been developed, which are better tolerated, which are better retained, which do not have the expulsion risk or the side effects of some of the larger bulky earlier devices," Davis told the committee. He talked about 300 young women who had never had children in whom he had inserted IUDs. (In his 12-month study, however, only 51 of the 640 women had never had children.)

Young unmarried women were particularly heartened by that statement. Thoroughly scared now by the Pill—and equally scared by the thought of getting pregnant—they wanted a device, a drug, anything, that would give them safe and effective protection against pregnancy. Davis was telling them that protection could be found in the IUD. For most women abortion was not an option. It would be three years before the Supreme Court would hand down its ruling in Roe v. Wade, affirming a woman's right to have an abortion in the first trimester of pregnancy.

Any concern about the safety of IUDs was brushed aside by Davis at the hearings. "I think that you can safely state that the major hazards of the use of an intrauterine device are related to the technical act of insertion," he said, "and that if you carry out technical precautions, it carries less risk than a smallpox vaccination which can under unusual circumstances lead to meningitis and death."

Davis also left unsaid something the Senators would no doubt have found very interesting—something that would have given an entirely different perspective to Davis' testimony. The matter was addressed at the very end of his testimony, when Davis was answering a series of questions from the committee's minority counsel, James Duffy.

MR. DUFFY: Doctor, while we are on the subject of intrauterine devices in our preparation for these hearings we became aware of the report that indicated that you had recently patented such a device. Is there any truth or substance to that report?

DR. DAVIS: I hold no recent patent on any intrauterine device. The Johns Hopkins University holds a patent on an intrauterine device that was developed in 1964 in a joint development venture together with the Ortho Research Foundation.

That particular device was a ring which was used for experimental purposes and has never been marketed, and I doubt ever will be marketed.

MR. DUFFY: You say you have—

DR. DAVIS: My name appears on a joint patent together with a Mr. Jones, and this patent is held jointly by the Johns Hopkins University for whom I am an employee, and by the Ortho Company. In the public interest this device was developed in 1964 and was the object of a patent application. This is not a marketed item and I doubt it ever will be.

MR. DUFFY: Then you have no particular commercial interest in any of the intrauterine devices?

DR. DAVIS: That is correct.

Of course, that wasn't correct. Davis had a 35 percent interest in the Dalkon Corporation, whose sole product was the Dalkon Shield.

Public reaction to the Pill hearings was quick and far-reaching. "Birth Pills Termed Still Experimental" was the front-page headline in the *New York Times*. In its January 26 edition, *Time* magazine ran a two-page article on the hearings, including a picture of Hugh Davis testifying.

The hearings served the needed purpose of warning women about the very real dangers of birth control pills. But in their rush to get off the Pill (and it is estimated that as many as one million women went off the Pill after the hearings), many women turned to the IUD. For some, it would prove just as treacherous.

With the demand for IUDs on the rise, Davis and Lerner were anxious to get their device on the mass market but were without the resources to do so. The Dalkon Corporation had no sales force and little money to advertise. The article in the *American Journal of Obstetrics & Gynecology* would certainly help, but it would take more than a single medical article to sell the device to doctors.

Their best chance at spreading the news about the Dalkon Shield was to set up demonstration booths at medical conventions. Such booths would be relatively inexpensive to put together. But who would operate these booths? Lerner wasn't a medical man, and Davis did not want to travel around the country openly peddling the device.

That's where Thad Earl came into the picture. Earl was a small-town general practitioner from Defiance, Ohio. He had no specialized training in obstetrics and gynecology, except for a couple of short hospital courses, but he was familiar with inserting IUDs by the end of 1969. And he hadn't been happy with them.

Lazar Margulies' Gynekoil was the first IUD Earl had inserted. He started inserting it after a salesman came around and gave him a package of 50. Earl had also prescribed the Lippes Loop and the Saf-T-Coil. But his patients had bad results with all three of these IUDs—bleeding, cramping, expulsion, and a high pregnancy rate, especially with the Gynekoil. Many of his patients were getting pregnant because they did not know their IUDs had been expelled.

Then, on November 3, 1969, Earl noticed a short article on page two in the *Defiance Crescent News* about Hugh Davis and the new IUD he was testing at Johns Hopkins University. Earl sent Davis a letter the next day. "I would be interested in coming to Baltimore to spend a couple of days with you and/or your clinic for instructions as to inserting of the IUD," he wrote. "I am most interested in this approach. I have a large gynecology practice, but up to the present time have been very dissatisfied with the IUDs on the market."

A blizzard forced Earl to cancel his first trip to the clinic, but early in December he flew to Baltimore where he met with Davis and watched the Johns Hopkins professor insert the device in a few of his patients. Earl himself was then allowed to try some insertions on Davis' patients. He liked the device—especially the 1.1 pregnancy rate which Davis was claiming for his IUD. Davis apparently failed to tell Earl about the extra pregnancies that had occurred after his study had officially ended, which had raised the pregnancy rate closer to three percent.

Earl was also impressed by the insertion technique for the Dalkon Shield. He liked the fact that the inserter stick resembled a uterine sound. It made him feel more secure placing the IUD into the uterus. Before he returned to Defiance, he ordered 48 Dalkon Shields over the phone from Lerner. The IUDs arrived at his Ohio office within a few days and Earl started inserting them immediately. One of his first patients was his wife. Earl continued to give his patients 1/120 of a gram of the anesthesia Atropine before inserting the Dalkon Shield, just as he had always done with the other devices. Unlike Hugh Davis, Earl did not recommend to any of his patients that they also use a spermicidal foam, jelly, or cream. Earl says Davis didn't tell him he had been making such recommendations to his patients.

Thad Earl wasn't content, however, to limit his involvement with the Dalkon Shield simply to using it in his medical practice. He saw, as he later put it, "a great future" for the Dalkon Shield, a future he wanted to be a part of. On New Year's Eve, less than three weeks after he began inserting Dalkon Shields in his patients, Earl flew to Connecticut to talk business with Lerner. Earl could offer the Dalkon Corporation what it needed—an enthusiastic physician with cash.

The company needed a medical director, someone who could be out front promoting the product to medical companies as well as physicians. For by this time, Lerner believed that the Dalkon Corporation would never be equipped to market the Shield effectively on its own. He wanted to sell the device to a large pharmaceutical company, one that could easily promote the Shield worldwide. His plan was to sell the device, but retain royalty rights for the Dalkon Corporation. Under the arrangement Lerner envisioned, Lerner, Davis, Cohn—and anyone else owning stock in the corporation—would always receive money from sales of the Shield. Yet even to sell the device to another company would take some promotion—and cash.

Earl says that Lerner first offered him a finder's fee of five percent of the Dalkon stock if he could find a purchaser for the Dalkon Shield and another five percent if he contributed $50,000 to the Dalkon Corporation. But this original offer was later dropped, and Lerner eventually agreed to give Earl 7.5 percent of the stock for his $50,000 and no finder's fee.

Davis did not seem to have been too pleased with Earl's addition to the Dalkon Corporation. An official with the pharmaceutical company that eventually purchased the Shield later said Davis appeared to consider Earl "a 'Johnny-come-lately' whose 'snake oil approach' would 'turn many people off.' " Davis told the official that he, Davis, would be able to reach people at the FDA, the World Population Council, and at various ob-gyn departments where Earl could not, but that Earl's "enthusiasm" would be useful at medical exhibits and among general practitioners.

Despite Davis' seeming disdain for Earl, the Ohio doctor joined the Dalkon Shield team. The interests in the device were now: Lerner, 50.87

percent; Davis, 32.38 percent; Cohn, 9.25 percent; and Earl, 7.50 percent.

The Dalkon Corporation had its medical director and the cash needed to begin promoting the product. All it needed now was a large company willing to buy them out. Earl sent letters to the major pharmaceutical companies—Upjohn, Eli Lilly, Parke-Davis, Meade Johnson, Abbott—to try and interest them in buying the Dalkon Shield. He also began manning technical booths at various medical conventions, such as the April 1970 International Obstetrics and Gynecology meeting in New York. The interest in the Shield, especially in the wake of the Pill hearings, was definitely there. Earl began to believe a sale was imminent.

While Earl traveled around the country looking for a buyer during the early part of 1970, Davis and Lerner were busy modifying the Shield's design. In his 12-month study, Davis had used only one size of the Dalkon Shield, the size that was later known as the "standard" or "multiparous" size. ("Multiparous" refers to women who have given birth to at least one child.) But after the study, he and Lerner decided another, smaller size was needed for "nulliparous" women, or women who had never been pregnant. These women generally have smaller uterine cavities than those who have had children. They didn't need as large a device; in fact, a smaller device meant less chance of uterine rejection, for the uterus would be less likely to "notice" its presence and not try to expel it by contracting.

Lerner and Davis began to manufacture a smaller version of the Shield in March 1970, long after Davis' 12-month study was completed. The smaller version, therefore, was never part of that study. Davis acknowledges that he later observed a higher pregnancy rate of 2.6 percent in a small series of patients using the smaller, nulliparous Dalkon Shields. But, he quickly adds, too few women were involved in that informal study to make the results significant. He and Lerner, and later the pharmaceutical company that purchased the Shield, preferred to use the more favorable 1.1 percent statistic from Davis' original study when promoting both sizes of the device.

Davis and Lerner had also found that the Dalkon Shield had a tendency to split during removal; often, forceps would be needed to pull the broken device out. So the configuration of the plastic was changed to make it thinner, softer, and more flexible. Promotional materials for the device never mentioned these changes either. Davis insists that these changes would not have affected the outcome of his study—its pregnancy or expulsion rates, for example. But the question remains. How would he know without redoing the study with the altered version of the device?

Davis was interviewed a lot after the Pill hearings, and in those interviews he did mention another change in the Dalkon Shield—at least at first. It involved the addition of copper to the device, something that would later cause problems with federal regulators. "With the addition of copper, the shield device is virtually 100 percent effective in preventing pregnancy," Davis told *Good Housekeeping* magazine. Later Davis would insist he was only talking about experimental models of the Shield in these interviews, not the one that was marketed.

The Dalkon Shield used in Davis' study had barium sulfate in it. This mineral gave the Shield some, but apparently not enough, radiopaqueness (the ability to be seen on an X-ray). Doctors needed to be able to locate the device on an X-ray to make sure it hadn't perforated the uterus and moved into the pelvic cavity. Adding more barium sulfate would only have made it more likely the device would break in removal, so another metal had to be chosen to increase the radiopaqueness of the IUD.

Lerner considered adding zinc, but Davis suggested copper sulfate instead. At that time, studies originating from Santiago, Chile, had shown that adding a fine copper wire or copper dust to IUDs improved the contraceptive effectiveness of the devices—possibly by killing the sperm. Why not use copper in the Shield? Davis asked Lerner. It would solve the X-ray problem and it might improve the device's pregnancy rates.

The pregnancy rate was no doubt of concern to Davis, for his extended study had shown that the Shield was not superior to popular IUDs already on the market as he was claiming. And there was now yet another potential competitor in the IUD field—a T-shaped device wrapped with a thin copper wire. Designed by the Population Council, the Copper-T, as the device would later be called, was getting a lot of attention in the press. Its makers claimed it was 99 percent effective in preventing pregnancy.

So copper sulfate was added to the Dalkon Shield to improve its radiopaqueness and, it was hoped, its contraceptive effect. Lerner also threw in some metallic powdered copper to improve the melt flow index of the plastic, or the ability of the plastic to flow during molding and form better, stronger joints.

The Dalkon Shield now had so much copper in it that if left out in humid weather, it turned blue-green as the copper oxidized. Davis himself told Lerner he could taste the copper in the Shield by placing the device on his tongue. Lerner and Davis didn't bother to conduct new studies to see if the copper, or any of the other alterations for that matter, changed the effectiveness of the Shield.

They went to physicians and drug companies with Davis' original 12-

month study in hand, a study that showed a device that was considerably different than the one they were actually trying to sell.

It was this study that Thad Earl, standing in a booth at a May 1970 Bedford Springs, Pennsylvania, medical exhibition, handed to a salesman from a large pharmaceutical company who happened by.

The salesman, John McClure, worked for the A. H. Robins Company.

Prescription for Success

"Why doesn't the American public realize that a company that is over 100 years old wouldn't make a decision that could destroy it in a matter of minutes?"

—E. Claiborne Robins, Jr.,
President of the A. H. Robins Company,
as quoted in the *New York Times*, August 1, 1984.

The A. H. Robins Company that salesman, John McClure, worked for in 1970 had a long and proud history, a history that spanned three generations of a hard-working Virginian family.

It was a success story in the true tradition of the American Dream—a family of entrepreneurs, who turned a small business into a giant corporation through hard work and wise decisions. The dream started in 1866 when a young ex-Confederate soldier named Albert Hartley Robins opened an apothecary store at 523 North Second Street in Richmond, Virginia. Like other pharmacists of the day, Robins filled prescriptions with medicines he made himself in his store, using mortar and pestle, grinding mills, balances, and hundreds of herbs and powders. He also concocted some of his own prescriptions, which he sold directly to his customers.

One of these prescriptions was the Robins Cascara Compound, patented pills that Albert recommended for "Indigestion, Dyspepsia & Obstinate Constipation." Albert sold the compound over-the-counter, advertising occasionally in local newspapers to bring buyers into his store. His son, Claiborne, soon recognized an even more effective way to sell the product—directly to doctors. He started his own business, separate from his father's, but with the same name—the A. H. Robins Company.

Claiborne made the rounds of doctors' offices, selling the physicians on the merits of his product. Then he took his orders back to his office above his father's store where the pills were packaged and shipped. Soon, Robins Cascara Compound became the leading product of its kind east of the Mississippi River—much to the surprise of Albert Robins, who still frowned on the idea of promoting directly to doctors. He thought there was no future in it.

Claiborne died in 1912 of heart disease. His father (who died 23 years later at the age of 92) kept the apothecary store running for a few more years, but Claiborne's business—selling the Robins Cascara Compound to doctors—declined. It would have folded altogether if it hadn't been for the tenacious efforts of Claiborne's widow, Martha, who kept the business going on a shoestring for 21 more years; until her son, E. Claiborne, graduated from pharmacy school.

At first E. Claiborne was reluctant to follow in his father's and grandfather's footsteps. At one time he had a vague notion of becoming a teacher. But he adapted quickly to the pressures of the business world, turning what was once a small single-product business into a pharmaceutical giant. When E. Claiborne took over the A. H. Robins Company in 1933, the company had three employees (including his mother) and total sales of only $4,800. Fifty years later, in 1983, the company would have more than 6,000 employees and total sales of half-a-billion dollars.

E. Claiborne started modestly enough, borrowing $2,000 from a Richmond bank. He then went out on the road to try and sell the Robins Cascara Compound to doctors, just as his father had done. But after two months in the Washington, D.C., area, E. Claiborne realized that the company wasn't going to survive on the compound alone. He went back to Richmond to try and come up with a few new products.

While reading a medical journal, E. Claiborne learned about the advantages of combining belladonna alkaloids and phenobarbital to calm a spasmodic, or irritated, bowel. That gave him the idea for Donnatal, an antispasmodic drug that quickly became—and remains—one of A. H. Robins' best-selling products. "We based [Donnatal] on this magazine article, then used the magazine article to promote it," E. Claiborne explained years later in a corporate promotional brochure.

Armed with Donnatal and two other new products, E. Claiborne took to the road again, visiting doctors from Virginia to Texas in his Model A Ford, letting them know about the Robins name and products. For a long time, he paid himself only $10 a week. The hard work and self-sacrifice paid off. By 1942, annual sales had reached $100,000, enough to allow Robins to let others do the selling while he stayed in Richmond to run the business.

And the business had only just begun to boom. In 1949, A. H. Robins added three more formulated drugs (drugs that combine more than one ingredient) to their product line: Robitussin (the well-known cough preparation), Pabalate (an anti-rheumatic drug), and Entozyme (a drug designed to aid digestion). They were all good sellers. Within one year, sales doubled from one million to two million dollars.

"Our product strategy was to select therapeutic areas where there was a great market," E. Claiborne recalled. "We naturally felt that since we had limited resources it would be silly to go into a limited market area. So we concentrated on the areas where there was a large demand, such as gastrointestinal disturbances (Donnatal); and arthritic conditions (Pabalate); and coughs (Robitussin)."

Two years later, with business expanding, the company broke ground for a new building on Cummings Drive in north Richmond. It included a plant as well as offices. The company had been using the University of Richmond's laboratories to formulate its drug products. It now wanted its own research and development facilities.

New drugs were continually added to the product line: Robaxin (a muscle relaxant that was the company's first patented product), Dimetapp (an antihistamine and decongestant), Donnagel (an antidiarrheal), and Dopram (a respiratory stimulant). Robaxin was one of the company's first non-formulated or "single-entity" drugs. And Dimetapp was one of the first drugs Robins licensed from another drug company.

During the 1940s and 1950s, it was relatively easy to get new drug products to market. But in the early 1960s, stricter amendments to the Food and Drug Act were passed, making it more difficult to get new drugs approved. This was especially true of formulated drugs. The safety and efficacy for each active component of the drug had to be proven—an expensive and time-consuming proposition.

Under the new rules, pharmaceutical companies became edgy about the future of their industry. A. H. Robins was no exception.

"We felt that if the pharmaceutical industry ever came to a point where it was not as profitable, or its ability to operate were hampered, it would be good to be in other areas," recalled E. Claiborne.

Many pharmaceutical companies went into cosmetics. But selling make-up is quite different from selling medicines, and some of these companies later divested themselves of their cosmetic acquisitions when they found they didn't know what to do with them. E. Claiborne, on the other hand, decided to stick for the time being with a product sold primarily in drugstores. He bought the Morton Manufacturing Corporation, the firm that manufactured Chap Stick lip balm. Four years later and more confident, the company expanded even further by purchasing the Polk Miller Products Corporation, producers of the Sergeant's pet-care line, and Parfums Caron, a French perfume maker. Today, one-third of A. H. Robins' business is in non-pharmaceutical areas.

Diversification was not the only milestone A. H. Robins passed in 1963. It was also the year sales topped $50 million and the year of its first public offering of stock. Two years later, on May 6, 1965, A. H. Robins was listed on the New York Stock Exchange. E. Claiborne was on the floor of the Exchange when the first 100 stocks were sold.

The days of peddling his grandfather's patented medicine from the front seat of a Model A Ford were long gone. E. Claiborne was now sitting atop a very large corporation, with offices worldwide. The company even had its own research and development program, although its budget and staff lagged far behind Eli Lilly, Upjohn, and other leaders of the industry. E. Claiborne still preferred to buy or license products already developed elsewhere.

Although the A. H. Robins name wasn't as well known in the late 1960s as those of some of the large drug companies, it was well-respected. Part of its image stemmed from astute public relations. It courted doctors, especially young doctors who had yet to make allegiances to particular products, by quietly stroking their egos. For 11 years, from 1959 to 1970, the company ran a very successful series of double-page ads in medical journals that pictured "memorable moments in the education and training of medical students." In one of these "Doctor of Tomorrow" ads, a young, handsome physician is pictured with a stethoscope around his neck and the caption reads: "The man said Doctor, and the man meant me."

During the 1960s, the company also sponsored dinners for hospital resident physicians and interns. "In those days, there weren't any folks screaming about conflict of interest or buying the doctor," E. Claiborne recalled. "Of course, that never occurred to us because we didn't see how anybody could ever think that one meal and a drink would buy anybody. Today, we are in a different climate. You have people screaming and, of course, the residents and interns receive much higher salaries . . . So these dinners would not have the impact today that they had then because then they were really appreciated."

A. H. Robins has always made much of its benevolence. In 1969,

E. Claiborne donated $50 million worth of A. H. Robins stock to his alma mater, the University of Richmond. (A year earlier *Forbes* magazine had listed Robins as one of the 66 wealthiest men in America.) At the time it was reported to be the largest single bequest to a university. A decade earlier, the company was featured in *Life* magazine for closing up shop and taking all its employees on an all-expense paid trip to Cuba. In one photograph of the event, E. Claiborne is seen being transported upon the shoulders of his happy employees.

But perhaps the greatest factor in Robins' successful image has been the reputation of its products and the hard work of its salesmen.

In 1970, E. Claiborne was 60 years old and getting close to retirement. His son, E. Claiborne Jr. had recently graduated from business school, joined the firm, and was already being shuffled from department to department, getting thoroughly groomed for the eventual take-over of the company's presidency.

Then along came an article from a medical journal—much like the article E. Claiborne had read all those years earlier when he first started searching for new medicines to sell. It spoke in glowing terms of a new medical product, a superior IUD.

That article led to one of E. Claiborne's final acquisition decisions for A. H. Robins. It was a decision he would later deeply regret.

John McClure was known at A. H. Robins as a placid person, a man who seldom got excited about anything. But he got very excited about the Dalkon Shield. It seemed to the salesman that the doctors at the May 1970 Bedford Springs, Pennsylvania, convention were spending more time at the Dalkon Shield booth than at any other.

McClure spent an evening looking over Hugh Davis' study and the other materials Thad Earl had given him before returning to the Dalkon booth to talk with Earl again. He asked Earl if the Dalkon Corporation—or more important, the Dalkon Shield—was for sale.

"Yes," said Earl, "but we're already actively negotiating with a company." He told McClure that Upjohn had offered the Dalkon Corporation $500,000 plus a six percent royalty interest in future sales of the Shield.

"If A. H. Robins can beat Upjohn's offer," said Earl, "we'd be willing to listen."

A week later, Earl got a call from Roy Smith, A. H. Robins' director of product planning. He told Earl that his company was very interested in the Shield and that he—Smith—would like to visit Defiance, Ohio, for a closer look at the device.

"Sure," said Earl. "I suggest, however, that you bring with you an ob-gyn specialist. Someone who could be impartial."

Smith agreed. He invited John Board, an ob-gyn specialist at the Medical College of Virginia (MCV) in Richmond, to make the trip. Board's wife, Ann, worked for A. H. Robins. But Board had to cancel at the last minute when Ann became ill, and he suggested that a colleague of his at MCV, Dr. Edward Davis, go in his stead.

Ed Davis (no relation to Hugh) stood squarely in the middle of the road when it came to IUDs. He thought they were a very good method of contraception, but not as a first choice for women who had never had children. He believed the consequences of infection—never having a child—presented too great a risk for these women. Yet he was interested in this new IUD that was being touted as safe for all women. He agreed to make the trip.

Ed Davis, Roy Smith, and Dr. Fred Clark, A. H. Robins' medical director, boarded a chartered plane early on the morning of May 28, 1970, and flew to Defiance. Smith explained to Davis that in addition to having him evaluate the Dalkon Shield, A. H. Robins was interested in having his opinion on the broader potential for IUD use overseas.

Earl was an enthusiastic salesman, but he made as poor an impression on Ed Davis as he had on Hugh Davis. He struck Ed Davis as a man who was very taken with his own importance, and who thought he was terribly clever for having bought into the Dalkon Shield. Earl kept reassuring the visiting party that his enthusiasm for the Shield was not in any way colored by his financial interest in the device. "I'm an honest man," he told them. "I am already making too much money to be bought off."

Davis decided he would have to separate the device from its salesman and make a judgment on the Shield in spite of his opinion of Earl. While Clark and Davis (but not Smith) watched, Earl inserted Dalkon Shields in eight women during the span of a single morning. Earl explained the protocol he used for insertions. First, he requested his prospective IUD patients to come for the insertion while they were menstruating. Not only could he then be sure they weren't pregnant, but he believed it would make spotting and cramping less noticeable. Second, he gave the women a local anesthetic and, if they seemed particularly tense, a tranquilizer as well. Finally, he had each woman lie down on the examining table where he would examine her, clean her cervix, sound the uterus to determine its depth, and insert the IUD.

After watching Earl insert the device, Davis tried his hand at a couple. He was very impressed, especially with the way the Shield was inserted. He felt the Shield's inserter stick gave him more control over where the device was placed in the uterus than the "soda straw" inserters of other popular IUDs then on the market.

"If the statistics hold up," he told Smith, referring to Hugh Davis' 12-month study, "then this device would be a significant advance for IUDs." He later repeated this message to other senior officials at A. H. Robins, stressing again that Hugh Davis' study was the major factor in his favorable opinion of the Shield. No one at A. H. Robins ever told the Richmond doctor that Hugh Davis, like Thad Earl, had a financial interest in the Dalkon Shield. If he had known that, Ed Davis says now, he would have been very skeptical of the study's findings. As it was, Davis asked for several boxes of Shields to take home with him to Virginia, where he began using them almost immediately.

During the Defiance trip, Earl and Smith met alone in the den at Earl's home. Smith told Earl that if A. H. Robins bought the Shield, the company would be interested in hiring Earl as a consultant. Earl told Smith that A. H. Robins better act quickly, for the deal with Upjohn was ready to be closed. Less than a week later, Earl was invited down to Richmond to make his final sales pitch to some of the higher-ups at A. H. Robins. After being ushered into the company's board room, Earl showed the A. H. Robins people a silent 8-mm film he and Lerner had made of him inserting the Shield in a patient. (During preparation for the film, Earl had let Lerner, who had no medical training whatsoever, insert the Shield into one of his patients. Both men insist they had the patient's consent.)

The film had been spliced together from 16-mm footage taken in Earl's office, giving it a grainy, amateurish look. But with Earl's extemporaneous narration, the film took on the aura of authority. Earl was particularly proud of the part where he inserted the Shield in a uterus that had been removed during a hysterectomy; he thought it helped doctors see how snugly the device fitted in the uterus.

The film was titled "The Dalkon Corporation Presents the Dalkon Shield Protocol." Yet nowhere in the film was Earl shown giving a patient an anesthetic or a tranquilizer, although this was often part of his protocol when inserting Shields. (The woman patient, however, noticeably tightened her leg muscles at the moment the Shield was inserted. As no sound recording was made of the insertion and the woman's face is not seen, it's not known whether she also cried out in pain, as so many other women later testified they did.) Nor was it suggested as part of the protocol that doctors recommend contraceptive foam or gel to their patients during part of their monthly cycles, as Hugh Davis had sometimes done. The favorable figures from Davis' study, however, do appear in the film.

Continuation rate, 94 percent; medical removals, two percent; pregnancy rate, 1.1 percent.

After showing the film to the A. H. Robins officials, Earl answered questions about his experience with the Shield. He said that during the seven months he had been inserting the Shield, his patients had reported no pregnancies, no expulsions, and no removals. The presentation went well. Earl flew back to Defiance, confident that his pitch had made an impression on the A. H. Robins officials.

A couple of days later, several people from A. H. Robins, including Roy Smith, made a trip to Stamford, Connecticut to take a closer look at the Dalkon Corporation. Lerner gave Smith the names of doctors around the country who had been using the Shield, including two who were in the midst of conducting studies on the Shield's effectiveness. A. H. Robins wanted to ask them about their experience with the device.

By this time, A. H. Robins was very interested in purchasing the Shield. It wasn't the first time the company had considered purchasing an IUD. Company officials say they thought about buying another IUD during the mid-1960s, but the purchase was never made. None of these officials remembers, however, which device was under consideration or why the deal fell through.

The Dalkon Shield was another matter. By the time it came to A. H. Robins' attention, several of the company's pharmaceutical competitors, most notably the Ortho Pharmaceutical Company (Lippes Loop) and Schmid (Saf-T-Coil), had carved out nice niches for themselves in the IUD market. Sales of IUDs had more than doubled since 1966. And after the Pill hearings, it seemed that sales were destined to climb even more—especially if an IUD could be successfully sold to women who had never had children.

The Dalkon Shield looked to be a smart purchase.

"It seemed to be a device that had certain advantages over competitive devices," recalls Dr. Jack Freund, who as vice-president of A. H. Robins' medical department was the company's highest-ranking medical official in 1970. Freund says, however, that the Shield received no special treatment from the A. H. Robins Company during the acquisition stage. "The Shield was just another new product proposal," he says. "We handled it as we would any other product."

William Zimmer, however, saw it in a slightly different light. Zimmer was A. H. Robins' executive vice-president and chief operating officer at the time. (Later, he would become the company's president, breaking briefly the succession of the Robins' family members to that post.) "I thought it would show a versatility on our part to move into an area that showed more sophistication," Zimmer recalls. He says he never considered the Dalkon Shield a "large volume product" that would make the company large sums of money.

"I looked on this [as] a prestige product dealing with the greatest social problem—overpopulation," he says. Zimmer admits, however, that he did not have a longstanding concern about overpopulation. His concern started with the Dalkon Shield.

For a company looking into a product on which it didn't expect to make much money, A. H. Robins certainly generated a flurry of meetings—and memos—on the subject. But, then, Zimmer says the company didn't want Upjohn to beat them to the purchase.

On June 8, 1970, Oscar Klioze, director of A. H. Robins' pharmaceutical research and analytical services, contacted Lerner to ask him some technical questions about the Dalkon Shield. Through his conversation with Lerner, Klioze discovered that Lerner and Davis had not conducted any formal stability or accelerated aging tests on the Shield. In other words, no tests had been done to see if the Shield would deteriorate while in the uterus. If it did deteriorate, the device could break apart during removal. A dilation and curettage (D and C) operation would then be required to remove the broken parts left in the uterus. Although a D and C is a relatively quick and simple operation, it often must be done in a hospital and with a general anesthetic. Doctors and, of course patients, would want to know if the device they were using was prone to deterioration.

Klioze also learned that the plastic used in the device had been cleared by the FDA for use in the packaging of meat, but not for implantation in humans. Klioze wrote a memo about his conversation with Lerner, which he forwarded to five A. H. Robins officials, including Smith and Freund.

That same day, June 8, Fred Clark went to Baltimore to talk with Hugh Davis about the Shield, to check the data from his 12-month study, and to see if there were any "red flags" that A. H. Robins should consider before making a decision about purchasing the Shield. He found Davis to be "matter-of-fact" and "not overtly enthusiastic"—apparently not an eager promoter of his product. Davis was talkative, Clark recalled, "but seemingly guarded in glorifying the Dalkon Shield and in volunteering information germane to the Dalkon Company. Most information [was] elicited by questions—on a couple of points, he suggested that information be obtained from Lerner, only to later come through with the answer."

Despite Davis' reticence, Clark gathered a lot of information during his visit; information he wrote down in a confidential three-page memo that, like Klioze's memo, was circulated to several top-ranking officials at A. H. Robins. Later, that memo would come back to haunt the A. H. Robins Company, for it showed that even before purchasing the Dalkon Shield, the company knew that the figures Hugh Davis had presented in his 12-month study were wrong.

"Davis' first paper on his first-year experience mentions 640 insertions with five pregnancies," wrote Clark. "However, data given me for first 14 months (Sept. '68–Nov. '69) covers 832 insertions with 26 pregnancies." Thus, A. H. Robins knew that the Dalkon Shield had a disappointing 3.1 percent pregnancy rate, making the device inferior rather than "superior" to other competitive devices and oral contraceptives. Yet no attempt was made to inquire further into Davis' findings. Clark looked at only a fraction—six or eight—of Davis' patient sheets (the place where specific data on each woman's experience with the Shield was recorded). And A. H. Robins' own biostatistician, Lester Preston, was never asked to review Davis' 14-month data to determine the Shield's real pregnancy rate.

A. H. Robins claims the Clark memo was all a mistake, a matter of bad penmanship. "[The memo] was handwritten and Fred Clark wrote in Sanskrit," says one A. H. Robins official. "It defies description, his handwriting." Clark's secretary, says the official, simply misread his numbers when she typed up the memo the following day.

That explanation seems strained at best, however, in view of another memo that appeared only a few days later. On June 11, 1970, Jack Freund wrote a memo of his own in which he stated that Davis' one-year follow-up period for his study was not long enough "to project [pregnancy figures] with confidence to the population as a whole." Lerner had told him, Freund added, that Davis' pregnancy rate for the Shield was actually higher when a longer follow-up period was considered—2.3 percent rather than the reported 1.1 percent. (Where Lerner got the figure of 2.3 percent is unknown; he later said he could not remember telling Freund about a higher pregnancy rate.)

The higher figure didn't bother Freund, for 2.3 percent was still a lower pregnancy rate than for other popular IUDs on the market. Freund does acknowledge, however, the "need for continuing the research effort initiated by Dr. Davis and Mr. Lerner . . . to support the effectiveness and safety of this device." This need "should be emphasized," he stressed.

Besides visiting with Davis and Lerner, the company also reviewed the yet-to-be-completed studies of two California doctors. And it conducted a few informal telephone interviews with various other physicians around the country who had been using the Shield since the Dalkon Corporation began marketing it in late 1969 or early 1970 (the exact date is in dispute). Some of these names were those given to Smith by Lerner. "No severe complications were reported," concluded one memo on these calls, "but it is important to note that experience with the Dalkon Shield in all physicians contacted was limited to a matter of months."

So, on the basis of a few doctors' limited use of the Shield and on the basis of only one completed—and questionable—study conducted by a doctor who had a financial stake in the study's outcome, A. H. Robins purchased the patents and rights to the Dalkon Shield.

A. H. Robins had no experience in the contraceptive field, nor did it have an ob-gyn specialist on staff. In fact, up until the Bedford Springs medical exhibition less than a month earlier, the company had never seriously considered marketing a contraceptive.

Now, of course, that had changed. A. H. Robins had big plans for the Dalkon Shield.

The Dalkon Corporation sold the Shield to A. H. Robins rather than Upjohn simply because Robins made a better offer—$750,000 cash plus 10 percent royalties payable to the four Dalkon Corporation shareholders (Davis, Lerner, Earl, and Cohn). A. H. Robins further fattened the pot by hiring Earl, Davis, and Lerner as consultants. Earl was signed on at an annual salary of $30,000, Davis at $20,000, and Lerner at $12,500.

The Dalkon Corporation, with its meager marketing attempts, had sold around 27,000 Shields. A. H. Robins, of course, hoped to sell millions of the device. But it would be six months later, January 1971, before its national marketing campaign would get under way. In the meantime, the Shield continued to be assembled, packaged, and shipped under Lerner's supervision from a small, two-story factory building in Stamford, Connecticut. Profits began to accrue to A. H. Robins, however, within days of the purchase. The Dalkon Corporation sold the device at cost to A. H. Robins, around 35 cents each. A. H. Robins then sold them to doctors for around $4 each.

Not everyone with the A. H. Robins organization was pleased that the company had purchased the Shield. Three months after the device was bought, George E. Thomas, vice-president of A. H. Robins' international division, expressed his concerns about the Shield in a "Personal & Confidential" memo to William Zimmer.

"I worry that we seem to have no present or past R&D [research and development] effort on contraception and contraceptive methods," Thomas wrote, ". . . I worry about the fact that we have no market knowledge or experience in our company, and we are prepared to learn on the job."

His concerns went unheeded.

Almost immediately after A. H. Robins purchased the Shield, Davis and Lerner began pressuring the company to change the design of the device. Davis was especially unrelenting on this point. At one point he called Richmond "and got several people upset with his insistence that the Shield design be modified soon," according to a memo written by Bob Nickless, an A. H. Robins product management coordinator.

Davis was particularly concerned that the part of the Shield to which the nylon tail was attached was not strong enough and might break during removal. But he wanted other changes made on the Shield as well. On the standard-sized model, he wanted the width of the device reduced from 27 to 24 millimeters to make it easier to insert and remove and to reduce cramping and bleeding; he wanted the central membrane thinned to make the Shield more flexible and to allow it to stay inside the uterus longer; and he wanted the fins made more "bat-shaped" (that is, fatter at the tips and slightly rounded)—again for easier insertion and greater tolerance. On the small-sized model, Davis also wanted the fins rounded and blunted so as not to damage tissue during insertion.

At first A. H. Robins was reluctant to make any changes that might make the Shield less effective. "The matter of rounding fin tips and narrowing the width of the multiparous causes me concern on a logical basis since without clinical study we would have no way of knowing if such changes, although seemingly minor to Dr. Davis, would result in a greater expulsion rate and perhaps in other less than favorable results," wrote Nickless. Despite these concerns, however, A. H. Robins, as the Dalkon Corporation had done before it, went ahead with the changes—and with promoting the newly-designed device using the figures from Davis' 12-month study. The new Dalkon Shield, however, was now significantly different in shape and size than the one Davis had tested.

It was also significantly different in composition, for Lerner and Davis had added copper to it since the 12-month study. Roy Smith knew this and it concerned him. In fact, it had concerned him even before A. H. Robins bought the Shield. In a June 10, 1970 memo to C. E. Morton, an A. H. Robins general manager, Smith expressed his doubts about marketing a product so dissimilar to the one Davis had studied. A copy of the memo was also sent to Ernest Bender, vice-president of the A. H. Robins administrative staff.

"At the luncheon yesterday," Smith wrote, "we discussed the possible implications of utilizing the Davis paper for promotional purposes, while marketing a device not identical in composition to that on which the paper was based . . . We have relatively limited information on the Dalkon Shield in terms of length of usage, overall cases published, etc. Even with this relatively limited total case history, the bulk of the experience to date and the bulk of the available data is on the shield made from the plastic with barium sulfate added, but without either copper or copper sulfate."

Smith also worried that patients wearing the copper Shield had not been followed up specifically to see if the copper sulfate was having a harmful effect on their uteri. "Copper salts are irritant and astringent," he wrote. "This would seem to me to indicate a danger of causing increased discomfort."

But Smith's "principal hang-up," as he called it, involved what he called "implied warranty."

"If we sell a doctor a device with no mention that the content of the material includes a copper salt which may contribute to the overall effectiveness, then it would seem clear that the doctor was buying a device and expecting the results to be attributable to that device. What troubles me is our implication to him—in the absence of 'full disclosure'—that a device is doing the job, whereas we would actually be selling a device to which we had added copper sulfate for the express purpose of getting a 'drug effect.' "

That "drug effect" was, of course, a contraceptive effect. Davis and Lerner had added copper sulfate for that express purpose, as Smith acknowledges in his memo.

A. H. Robins decided not to disclose the inclusion of copper in the Shield in its promotional materials. The company did, however, leave its salesmen with the strong impression that the Shield's copper had a contraceptive effect.

"In addition to the total surface area of [an IUD] which is in contact with the endometrium," noted a piece of training material handed out to the salesmen, "it has been shown that certain metal ions, specifically copper ions will enhance the effectiveness of the device . . . The Shield device was specifically engineered to provide maximal surface area contact with the endometrium, and copper sulfate has been incorporated into the plastic mix from which the Shield is molded."

Many salesmen took the hint and passed on to doctors the idea that the Shield's copper had a contraceptive effect—at least, they did at first. Later, when the FDA began to consider regulating IUDs that had a "drug effect," A. H. Robins carefully disengaged itself from any claims that the copper in the Dalkon Shield helped prevent conception. Although at that time the FDA was not regulating medical devices, such as IUDs, it did require that anything classified as a drug be tested for safety and efficacy before being marketed. If the Shield were to be classified as a drug, A. H. Robins would have to subject the device to expensive FDA-sanctioned tests. If the Shield failed those tests, the FDA could order it off the market.

But that part of the story would begin to unravel later. In the meantime, something else came up during discussions about design changes in the Shield, something that would play a major role in the Dalkon Shield story. It involved the tail string.

Sometime in June 1970, Win Lerner warned A. H. Robins officials that the Dalkon Shield's multifilament tail string had a wicking tendency and could carry potentially deadly bacteria to the uterus. He recommended finding a new material for the string. This warning was widely circulated among A. H. Robins officials in a Dalkon Shield "orientation report" written by Bob Nickless on June 29, 1970. "The string or tail situation needs a careful review since the present 'tail' is reported (by Mr. Lerner) to have a 'wicking' tendency," wrote Nickless. This memo was sent to 39 A. H. Robins officials.

Thus, six months before marketing the device nationally (and only three weeks after purchasing it), A. H. Robins knew that the multifilament string presented a potentially dangerous situation for the women who wore the Shield. Yet the company never conducted its own wicking studies on the multifilament string during the four years the Shield was on the market.

A. H. Robins insists, however, that the "careful review" Nickless called for in his memo was done. The job was assigned to Dr. Fletcher Owen, who, as A. H. Robins' director of medical services, was responsible for the Shield's labeling, advertising, and promotional materials.

"I examined the medical literature specifically and all of the learned treatises available . . . to see what the consensus was with respect to tailed versus tailless devices," Owen recalls. He says he found nothing in the literature to raise his concern about the Shield's string. But Owen also acknowledges that at the time he conducted his careful review he did not know the Shield had a multifilament tail string. He knew only that it was made of a nylon surgical suture material. Yet all the articles he consulted referred to the state-of-the-art "monofilament" tails. There was nothing

65

in the literature about multifilament ones, because they hadn't been used before.

With its "careful review" out of the way, A. H. Robins threw its efforts during the summer and fall of 1970 into putting together a massive marketing campaign, one that would soon make the Dalkon Shield the best-selling IUD in the country.

7

Selling the Shield

―――――――――

"But, after all, we are in business to sell the thing, to make a profit. I don't mean we're trying to go out and sell products that are going to be dangerous, fatal, or what have you. But you don't put all the bad things in big headlines."
　　　　　　　　—A. H. Robins official, quoted anonymously
　　　　　　　　in the *National Observer*, September 8, 1973.

In January 1971, A. H. Robins kicked off its national marketing campaign for the Dalkon Shield. It was a lavishly designed production, one of the most aggressive promotional campaigns in A. H. Robins' history.

"The need for a good initial show is imperative," stressed a preliminary market study prepared by the A. H. Robins marketing research department several months earlier. The campaign was first aimed at doctors—specifically general practitioners, osteopaths, and ob-gyn specialists. These were the doctors most likely to dispense contraceptives. But the preliminary market study warned that the device should not be pressed on a general practitioner or osteopath "who is just casually familiar with pelvic anatomy." It wasn't a concern about women's health that prompted that warning, however.

"Such sales," the report stated, "could be very detrimental to the establishment of this product. Complications are sometimes evaluated by number and severity and not why they came about. It would be to our advantage to keep our 'press' as good as possible until use is more widespread and the merits of our device better known. Once proven and accepted, complications in conjunction with use of the DALKON SHIELD would be far less damaging."

Less damaging to whom? A. H. Robins or the women who suffered those "complications"? The company already seemed more interested in possible damages to sales than in damages to the health of women.

A. H. Robins knew it might have an uphill battle selling its new IUD to doctors. Twenty-eight doctors had been surveyed for the marketing report, and their reactions had been "varied and inconsistent" at best.

"While many physicians felt that simplicity, flexibility and apparent ease of insertion would definitely be promotionally advantageous," noted the report, "others had serious reservations concerning the ability of the SHIELD to pass through the cervix without creating unnecessary pain and trauma . . . Several were appalled by what they considered the 'frightening' looks of the device and very concerned with the possibility of these fins tearing roughly into the uterus upon withdrawal . . . In some cases the rigidity of the inserter and its round tip were considered advantageous while others felt that rigidity would impede insertion in the severely introflexed or retroflexed uterus and that the tip increased the possibility of perforation."

Like other pharmaceutical companies, A. H. Robins relied heavily on its national network of salesmen, called "detailmen," to get out the word to doctors about the Dalkon Shield. In 1970, Robins had 560 detailmen, considered one of the best and most aggressive sales forces in the country. Their job was to "detail" doctors, hospitals, and other health care providers by visiting their offices and describing the company's products— just as E. Claiborne, Sr., had done himself back in the 1930s and 1940s. Rarely, however, did the detailmen take actual orders or deliver goods. Their role was strictly one of promotion.

Detailmen generally rely on information given them by their employer, and A. H. Robins' detailmen were no exception. For their first presentation of the Dalkon Shield to doctors, the company's detailmen were given an array of carefully designed materials. During the first few months of 1971 alone, A. H. Robins' detailmen disseminated 200,000 file cards (reference cards containing information about the Dalkon Shield for physicians to place in their own card index); 65,000 patient aid pads (pads with about 50 informational tear-out sheets for doctors to give to patients); 5,200 visual aid cards (full-color eight-page displays for the detailmen to use while talking with doctors); 80,000 reprints of Hugh Davis' February 1970 article from the *American Journal of Obstetrics & Gynecology*; 42,000 copies of a *Medical World News* article entitled "The Dalkon Shield May Carry the Day of IUDs"; and 80,000 copies of an article by Dr. Christopher Tietze, a well-known expert in the field of contraception. (Tietze's article had nothing to do with the Dalkon Shield, but it praised IUDs in general.)

File cards, visual aid cards, and other kinds of promotional material delivered directly to doctors are referred to as "labeling" in drug company parlance. Labeling also includes any information contained on the label or package insert of the product. Promotional material aimed at the medical community at large (for instance, an ad placed in a medical journal) is known as "advertising."

If a drug company uses false or misleading information in its labeling or advertising, or if a company fails to reveal material facts in these materials, the company could be found guilty of misbranding under federal law.

The Dalkon Shield file card (actually a set of cards given in a small folder to doctors for future reference) promoted the Shield as "the modern, sophisticated intrauterine device with a superior [there's that word again], rational design." It claimed the Shield prevented pregnancy "without producing any general effects on the body, blood or brain" and without disrupting normal menstrual periods. The card also claimed that the Shield was "well suited for nulliparous, as well as multiparous patients" and had "exceptional patient tolerance." Davis' findings—including the claim of a 1.1 percent pregnancy rate, which A. H. Robins now knew was false—were boldly superimposed on a chart compiled by Christopher Tietze that showed the comparative rates of other IUDs.

Comparing the Dalkon Shield data with Tietze's data was unfair and misleading, for the tests involved entirely different groups of women and quite different testing centers. Tietze's data, for example, involved 29 investigators and 31,000 women, figures that make Davis' test group of 640 women seem insignificant in comparison.

A source note to the chart on the Dalkon Shield file card referred to Davis and his *American Journal of Obstetrics & Gynecology* article. However, nowhere in the file card was it noted that Davis was receiving royalties from Shield sales and was a paid consultant to A. H. Robins, or that the Shields used by Davis in his test were substantially different than those sold by A. H. Robins. Nor was it noted anywhere on the file card that both Hugh Davis and Thad Earl gave many of their patients an anesthetic before inserting the Shield to reduce pain and cramping. The A. H. Robins protocol for insertion made no mention of an anesthetic; on the contrary, the company claimed the device could be easily inserted in "even the most sensitive woman."

The file card and other promotional materials also failed to tell the doctors to recommend contraceptive foam to their Shield patients for the first three months of use. Davis and Lerner had put this recommendation on the file card they had sent to doctors while the Dalkon Corporation was manufacturing the Shield. Although they restored it on a later card, A. H. Robins deleted it from their first file card, presumably because they feared that physicians might not purchase a device that required an additional contraceptive.

As is the general industry practice, warnings about the Shield appeared in small print on the final page of the file card. Doctors were cautioned that "sepsis may result from unclean technic" and "perforation may result from traumatic insertions." These statements clearly imply that any problems with the Shield would be the fault of the doctor, not the device's design. This would later become a major theme of the A. H. Robins defense as an avalanche of lawsuits came down upon the company.

In its first file card, for example, A. H. Robins stressed that with the Shield "correct insertion is simple and placement is accurate" due to a "combination of the superior shield design and an improved insertion technic [that] assures high fundal placement." In other words, the device's design assured that it would be placed high in the uterus, where it was believed to be most effective. Later, however, the company dropped this guarantee and instead asserted that doctors would have to strictly follow the insertion protocol to assure proper placement of the device in the uterus. Again, the implication was clear—if a woman became pregnant, it was the fault of the doctor, not the device.

The possibility of PID was not mentioned although A. H. Robins' competitor, the Ortho Pharmaceutical Company, had included a general warning about PID (although a very weak one) in its file cards for the Lippes Loop as early as 1965.

The message from A. H. Robins was clear in its file card—the Shield offered a "sure, safe, sensible contraception." Yet at the time it began its national campaign, A. H. Robins had no trained or experienced ob-gyn staff, nor had it completed any pre-market testing of the device, except for a 72-hour implantation in animals to test the plastic for irritation.

At least one A. H. Robins official, Fred Clark, was concerned about this lack of pre-market testing—or about the appearance of a lack of testing. Two-and-a-half months before the national marketing campaign, Clark complained in a memo circulated among several A. H. Robins officials that the company had no individual data forms documenting the use of either the old or new models of the Dalkon Shield. Such statistical or background information was needed to answer the requests for source material which were sure to come in from doctors and others once the product was heavily marketed.

"It appears desirable to HAVE SOME use documentation in our File," Clark wrote. "IN ADDITION, it appears desirable to obtain 'preliminary' comment from 1-2 other investigators regarding the use of the newly modified standard Shield . . . under the assumption that 1-2 month observations by [January 1, 1971] would be better than nothing. Therefore, please proceed to effect whatever arrangements are needed to get the new model into the hands of an investigator or two, as soon as possible." Brief "observations" by "an investigator or two" were apparently the extent of the A. H. Robins pre-market testing.

Most pharmaceutical companies, including A. H. Robins, are members of a powerful trade organization called the Pharmaceutical Manufacturer's Association (PMA). Members of the association are expected to adhere to its code of fair practices when promoting drug products. According to E. C. Robins, Sr., while the company believed that technically it was not bound to the code when promoting the Dalkon Shield because the Shield was a medical device rather than a drug, the company still felt ethically obliged to follow the code's tenets.

According to the PMA's 1967 code in place at the time, A. H. Robins began marketing the Shield, information concerning marketed drug products should be made available "promptly" to the medical profession and should be "complete and accurate." In addition to requiring a description of indicated uses or dosage recommendations for a product, the code required promotional communications to include complete information on side effects, precautions, warnings, contraindications (conditions or symptoms that make a particular treatment or procedure inadvisable), and effectiveness. The PMA code also insisted that statements used in the promotion of drug products be based upon substantial scientific evidence or other responsible medical opinion. "Claims are not to be ambiguous or stronger than the evidence warrants," the code stated.

At the time it began its national marketing campaign, A. H. Robins knew the effectiveness of the Shield was not the 1.1 percent pregnancy rate it was advertising. And it also knew that the tail string of the device posed potential dangers.

Warnings had come from outside as well as inside the company. In November 1970, one of the A. H. Robins detailmen wrote a letter to the company about a conversation he had had with a Detroit doctor whose "credentials are most impressive." The doctor told the detailman that A. H. Robins "does not have a superior IUD and is going to run into problems." He also charged that the company's "statistics (re. Dr. Davis)

71

are biased and he holds a very low opinion of Dr. Davis [and] Dr. J. T. Earl."

A. H. Robins apparently preferred to brush off these charges, rather than explore their validity.

The big send-off for the Dalkon Shield worked. Sales began to climb dramatically. A. H. Robins estimated that in January 1971, 29,000 Shields were inserted in women; six months later, in June, the monthly insertion rate had more than doubled to 66,000. The marketing campaign also seemed to have an impact on all IUD sales. In 1971, the total number of IUDs sold in the United States jumped by almost half-a-million, to 1,670,000.

The publication in September 1971 of an article and a book about the Shield boosted even further the sales of the device. The article, entitled "The Shield Intrauterine Device" was written by Thad Earl and published in *American Family Physician*, a medical journal. In it, Earl reported on his 15-month study of the Dalkon Shield, a study he had conducted on his patients in Defiance, Ohio, from December 1969 (the month he picked up his first Shields from Lerner) to March 1, 1971.

Earl reported that of the 536 Shield-wearers in his study, only two became pregnant, indicating a pregnancy rate of .5 percent. (A third woman in the study reported her pregnancy to Earl in mid-April; Earl considered this too long after his cut-off date of March 1 to be included in his findings.) He also reported that his continuation rate—the percentage of women who kept wearing the Shield—was 95.4 percent. These figures were even better than those Davis had reported more than a year earlier (a 1.1 percent pregnancy rate and a 94 percent continuation rate).

A. H. Robins helped Earl draft the article, and Lester Preston, A. H. Robins' biostatistician, performed the calculations for his findings. A. H. Robins' participation was not noted in the article, however, nor was it mentioned that Earl was a paid consultant to A. H. Robins and was a recipient of royalties for Dalkon Shield sales. After the article was published, Earl authorized A. H. Robins to buy reprints of it. Seventy-seven thousand copies were ordered and presumably distributed to doctors.

That same month, September 1971, Hugh Davis made an even bigger publishing splash with his new book on IUDs. The book was published by the Williams and Wilkins Company, a respected medical textbook publishing company based in Baltimore, and it received considerable attention from the popular press as well as from the medical profession.

The Intrauterine Device for Contraception, Davis' book, praised the IUD as a "superior birth control method because it uniquely combines medical safety, simplicity, long-term efficacy and reversibility." And which IUD is the most superior? The Dalkon Shield, of course.

In the book Davis never recommends the Dalkon Shield above other IUDs in so many words. But in every chart, graph, and analysis, the Shield is shown to be clearly superior. For example, in a chart comparing the "complications reported per 100 woman-years in first year of use for 10 major IUD's," no other IUD comes even close to Davis' reported total complication rate for the Shield (5.4 percent). The next best rate is given to the Ota Ring (16.9 percent) while the Shield's stronger competitors, the Lippes Loop and Saf-T-Coil, fared even more miserably—30.6 and 40.8 percent respectively.

Of course, these poor showings for all except the Shield raise another, even more basic question. How could Davis claim IUDs were a "superior" form of contraception when all of them, except for Davis' favored Shield, either failed to prevent pregnancy, were expelled by the uterus, or had to be removed for "medical" reasons in at least 15 of every 100 women who wore them? And why, with 30 to 40 percent of women having problems with the most popular devices, didn't doctors declare IUDs too dangerous and unreliable to be put into a woman's womb?

Nowhere in his book does Davis identify himself as the major source for the statistics on the Shield, or as co-inventor of the Shield, or as a paid consultant to the company that manufactures the Shield, or as someone who receives money for each Shield sold. Nor does he let his readers know that A. H. Robins reviewed the galleys of the book before it was published and reimbursed Davis for the artwork in the book. (In fact, according to Michael Pretl, a Baltimore attorney who talked with Davis' editor, Dick Hoover, shortly before Hoover's death, Davis didn't tell his publisher about any of these things, either.) The book looks and reads as if it were a purely objective review of IUDs.

Davis reported again in the book, as he had in his earlier article, that the pregnancy rate for the Shield was 1.1 percent, once again ignoring the results of his extended study. He also knew another investigator's pregnancy rates for the Shield were different than what he reported in his book. On page 46 of the book, Davis reports that in a study conducted in Santiago, Chile, only two of 400 Shield-users had become pregnant. In February 1971, however, seven months before publication of his book, Davis heard from the doctor conducting the study that there had been five pregnancies, indicating a pregnancy rate of 4.1 percent. Davis claims it was too late to change the figures for his book.

Davis was proud of his book; he bought 124 copies at his own expense, autographed them, and mailed them out to whomever he thought might be interested. (Later he hinted in a letter to Lerner that he thought either Lerner or A. H. Robins should reimburse him for the expense of this "promotional activity.") Davis suggested to A. H. Robins officials that the company buy the book in bulk and give copies to all its detailmen. A. H. Robins declined, although it did do some bulk buying for overseas use.

A. H. Robins didn't need the book for its American sales force in 1971 because the Shield was already selling well. And the company had other ways to ensure the detailmen sold the Shield—it applied heavy pressure on them to meet sales quotas, pressure enough to cause one regional manager to threaten his detailmen with their jobs. A telegram from this manager delivered a not-so-subtle message: "Northern Division will not be humiliated by a lack of Dalkon sales," read the telegram. "If you have not sold at least 25 packages of 8 then you are instructed to call me. Be prepared to give me your callback figures. No excuses or hedging will be tolerated, or look for another occupation."

From the beginning of the marketing campaign, the detailmen were instructed to stress data that showed the Shield to be safe for women who had never had children. "Positive data in this area expands the potential market significantly," stated the Shield's preliminary market study.

However, reports on sales soon were eclipsed by another, darker set of reports making their way to Richmond. Within weeks of the beginning of the promotional blitz for the Shield, A. H. Robins began hearing from doctors who were anything but impressed with this "superior" IUD. Some of the earliest complaints went to the very heart of the A. H. Robins campaign—doctors said they were unable to duplicate Davis' 1.1 pregnancy rate.

"I have a group of Ob-Gyn physicians who have been using the Dalkon Shield since March of 1970," wrote one Robins detailman based in Connecticut. "They have made 206 insertions of the devices up to February of this year. They have had 8 pregnancies attributed to 'the shield,' 4 multiparous and 4 nulliparous. I have gone over protocol, technique, etc. with them and fail to find [any] reason for their results . . . They think our figures are inaccurate and not based on enough cases. They say that 'the shield' is not better than the other IUD's on the market today."

On April 20, 1971, a letter arrived from a Canadian doctor with the same complaint:

"I have inserted 58 Dalkon Shields since May 6, 1970," wrote the doctor. "I first saw these shields at the World Congress in New York City in May and they appeared at that time to be an advance. Unfortunately, this is not so, as four pregnancies have developed in the 58 women." One of the women had had a spontaneous abortion; the Shield was found in the placenta.

Yet another letter went directly to Davis. "I have read your book, *The IUD*, and find it to be very interesting and helpful," a Maryland doctor wrote. "There is one thing that I cannot explain and that is why I have been having a high pregnancy rate with the Dalkon Shield in spite of the fact that we've been using the same technique you describe in your book. As a matter of fact, most of the colleagues in this area have stopped using the shield because the result has not been good at all. Could you suggest to me what improvements I should make in order to get your result as far as pregnancy is concerned?"

During the following months, as more and more doctors began to use the Shield, these complaints would mount—and mount and mount. On June 15, 1971, came a report of six pregnancies out of 12 insertions; on June 23, eight out of 250; on July 9, three out of 65; on July 23, six out of 180; on July 26, six out of 100; on August 30, 12 out of 300. Clearly, something was wrong.

In responding to these doctors, A. H. Robins began to make the recommendation that they had earlier decided to leave out of the promotional materials—the patient should use an additional contraceptive measure for the first three months after insertion. By the end of the year, the company was including that recommendation on the Shield's labeling.

As for the discrepancy between the pregnancy rate experienced by the doctors writing to A. H. Robins and that reported in the Dalkon Shield's promotional literature, A. H. Robins blamed it on "enlarged or relaxed uteri" or "variations in length of the cervical canal and the endometrial cavity." The problem, A. H. Robins seemed to be claiming, was not with the device, but with the women who were wearing it. Their anatomy wasn't right. Yet this was the IUD designed for the "average" uterus and promoted as "anatomically engineered for optimum uterine placement, fit, tolerance and retention."

Pregnancy wasn't the only concern of doctors using the Shield. Many doctors complained about the extreme pain their patients experienced during insertion of the device. One doctor wrote that the unfolding of the Shield in his patients' uteri startled and hurt them to such an extent that with each insertion he worried he had perforated the uterus. Another angry doctor wrote that he had inserted "thousands" of IUDs in his practice, but had found that the insertion of the Dalkon Shield to be "the most traumatic manipulation ever perpetrated upon womanhood."

Almost all other commercial IUDs at the time were long thin pieces of plastic that curled into their various shapes once they were inserted into the uterus. They were put into the uterus with a "soda straw" inserter that allowed the IUDs to slip through the cervix in their stretched-out forms. Dilation of the cervix was not required. Nor was much needed. The Dalkon Shield, on the other hand, was broad and flat and could not be folded or stretched to fit easily through the cervix. (Lerner later obtained a patent for a Shield with collapsible fins, but the design never left the drawing board.)

The Shield required tremendous force for insertion. A. H. Robins' own tests (conducted in 1973) showed that even the small nulliparous model required 10 times more force for insertion than the Lippes Loop. And when Ellen Preston, a staff physician at A. H. Robins, experimented with inserting the Shield into a plastic model of a uterus, she found that the model's cervix became partially unglued after several insertions and removals.

Removing the device was also an excruciating ordeal for many women, and their doctors complained to A. H. Robins about it. One doctor, after struggling to remove the Shield from a patient in his office, said he finally had to put the woman in a hospital and take out the device while she was under a general anesthesia. Another doctor complained of having difficulty removing the device from a patient who had become pregnant while wearing it. She eventually had to have a therapeutic abortion.

Preston conceded in her correspondence to one doctor that insertion of the Shield "is somewhat more difficult than insertion of other available IUDs," a concession that is in direct contradiction to A. H. Robins' promotional materials for the Shield. Preston also recommended that before inserting the device, the doctor give some of his patients Demerol (a painkiller), Atropine (a drug that protects against pain-induced cardiac arrest), and a paracervical block. These were the recommendations the Dalkon Corporation had made on its labeling for the Shield, but which had been dropped by the A. H. Robins Company.

In mid-July of 1971, six months after A. H. Robins began marketing the Shield, the company called a meeting of its medical experts, including Board, Clark, Owen, Nickless, Ellen Preston, and Lester Preston, to review doctor complaints about difficult insertions and removals and about the "undesirable rate of removal for pain and bleeding during one-two months." The experts decided at the end of the meeting that "while problems are recognized, the overall view is that we are not accumulating information suggesting that we have an 'inferior' product."

All of these complaints raised serious questions about the safety and efficacy of the Shield. But soon another group of reports started coming in from doctors describing an even more disturbing problem—PID. And the culprit appeared to be the device's wicking tail string—the very problem Lerner had warned A. H. Robins about three weeks after the company purchased the Shield.

One of the first hints of a problem came in a roundabout way, and from an odd source—Ortho. "What is our Dalkon 'string' made of?" asked an A. H. Robins detailman from California in a handwritten memo to the company's medical department. "Competition (Ortho) is telling my doctors that it will break, it will fray easily, and that it is 'multi-layered' so that the inner core acts as a wick to induce infection into the uterus." The memo was handmarked "Important, Please Rush" at the top.

Later, in another memo written like a script, a detailman described a conversation he had with a dissatisfied Connecticut doctor:

[DOCTOR]: "How many infections have you had with the Dalkon Shield?"

[DETAILMAN]: "None that I know of, why?"

[DOCTOR]: "I've had two that had to be removed because of infections."

[DETAILMAN]: "Who inserted them?"

[DOCTOR]: "Someone else from out of town."

[DETAILMAN]: "How long ago?"

[DOCTOR]: "Four to six months ago."

[DETAILMAN]: "Do you think the insertion was a clean insertion?"

[DOCTOR]: "Yes, the infection came four to five months later."

[DETAILMAN]: "Do you think the infection came from the Shield?"

[DOCTOR]: "I'm not sure, that's why I ask."

[DETAILMAN]: "Is it possible it may have been caused by something else?"

[DOCTOR]: "Yes, but I wonder if the Shield may have caused it."

[DETAILMAN]: "I will check with our medical department."

The detailman did check with the A. H. Robins medical department, specifically with Ellen Preston, a staff physician who had no training or experience in the ob-gyn field. In her job as project coordinator, Preston was expected to collect "adverse reaction" reports from doctors and respond to them.

Preston wrote to the doctor what she hoped would be a reassuring letter. "Reports of infections in Dalkon Shield patients have been rare," she told him. "In several large studies involving approximately 2,000 patients there were few if any cases of PID."

She didn't tell the doctor that those studies were grossly inadequate—and that A. H. Robins knew they were inadequate.

Nor did she tell him of Wayne Crowder and his wicking experiment.

These were secrets A. H. Robins would keep to itself for many months to come.

8

A String Attached

*"I told him that I couldn't in good conscience not say
something about something that I felt could cause infections.
And he said that my conscience didn't pay my salary."*
—Wayne Crowder, a quality control supervisor
for the Dalkon Shield, March 27, 1981.

One afternoon in the middle of March 1971, 34-year-old Wayne
Crowder walked through the Chap Stick Company's plant in Lynchburg,
Virginia, and noticed two women workers tying strings to small plastic
discs that looked to Crowder like fishing lures.

"What are those things?" he asked the employees, pointing to the
plastic objects in their hands.

"Contraceptive devices," the women answered.

Immediately, Crowder went to Julian Ross, his superior at Chap Stick,
to tell him that a contraceptive device was being assembled in the plant
and to find out if any provision had been made for its quality control.
Since 1968, Crowder had been Chap Stick's quality control supervisor. It
was his job to make sure the quality of the company's products met
established standards and were safe and as intended for consumer use.

Ross wasn't surprised by Crowder's news of the device. "I've been
meaning to speak to you about it," he told Crowder. He then explained
that the device—the Dalkon Shield IUD—had been acquired by A. H.
Robins, Chap Stick's parent company. A. H. Robins had assigned its
Lynchburg subsidiary the job of assembling and packaging the device, a
job that had previously been done in Stamford, Connecticut. It was

expected that, because of savings in labor and other costs, the move to Lynchburg would bring the manufacturing bill for each Shield down to 25 cents from 35 cents—a substantial savings. Chap Stick would have partial responsibility for quality control over the product, Ross continued, and Crowder would be in charge of that quality control.

Crowder was astonished. The product was already being assembled at Chap Stick (the first shipment from Lynchburg was scheduled for May), and no quality control procedures had yet been established. A. H. Robins hadn't even sent over its quality control manual for the device.

Crowder went to work at once, familiarizing himself with the Shield. He requested the Shield's quality control manual, and after several days, finally got it. Crowder felt that the manual was deficient; it did not provide for adequate quality control procedures, and it needed to be rewritten.

At the end of March, Crowder flew to Connecticut to see how the Dalkon Corporation had been manufacturing the device, and to talk with Win Lerner. As Lerner took him on a tour of the Dalkon operations, Crowder found himself particularly drawn to one aspect of the device— the string. It was different from any string he had ever seen before. In configuration, it roughly resembled a strand of electrical wire, for it was a bundle of plastic fibers enclosed by a sheath, much like the insulation on a wire.

Crowder asked Lerner why he had chosen that particular string, and Lerner explained that a solid, or monofilament, string would have been too stiff.

Then Crowder asked why he just didn't use a simple braided string, without the sheath. The sheath, Lerner explained, was to keep the string dry so body fluids containing bacteria could not migrate from the vagina into the uterus.

When asked how the string could be kept dry inside when both ends of the string were cut and open, Lerner explained to Crowder that the two knots in the string served as a barrier to the migration of water.

Crowder pondered this a moment, then took out his cigarette lighter, flicked it on, and passed a piece of the string through the flame. The string's end melted and shriveled into a small bead. Beading might be a better way of sealing the string from moisture and bacteria, Crowder suggested, and it might also solve the "male sensitivity" problem.

Earlier, Lerner had told Crowder about complaints A. H. Robins had been receiving from the sexual partners of women wearing the Shield. The end of the string that protruded from the cervix into the vagina was painful to some men during intercourse. A. H. Robins considered this a significant problem and was looking for a solution. Beading the end of the string would make it round and blunt—and less obtrusive, Crowder told Lerner.

Lerner said he would think about the suggestion and Crowder didn't pursue it with him any further. But Crowder considered the open-ended sheath to be a serious design flaw in the product, an open invitation to infection. On his return from Connecticut, Crowder shared his concerns about the string with Ross. Ross told Crowder that the design of the device wasn't his responsibility and to leave it alone.

But Crowder wouldn't leave it alone. As quality control supervisor, he felt any flaws in the string very definitely came under his responsibilities. He immersed himself in all the literature he could find on contraceptives and IUDs, borrowing books on the subject from a friend who was a doctor.

In the meantime, Chap Stick hired more people to assemble and package the Shield. Their job was to tie the strings onto the device, mount the device onto the inserter stick, then mount the device and the stick onto a display card. They then put all of this into a plastic bag, which was sealed and sent off to another site, where the entire packet was sterilized.

From the beginning, workers complained of sore hands from pulling the strings during the tying operation. But by far the biggest complaint was the production pressure. Thanks to A. H. Robins' very successful advertising campaign, Dalkon Shields were being sold faster than they could be produced.

The first shipment from Chap Stick went out in May 1971. There were problems with the string from the start. The sheath was being stripped and mashed during the tying process, creating tiny holes in the sheath just below the knot that attached the string to the bottom rim of the device.

In June, Crowder examined under a microscope samples of Shields ready to be shipped from the Chap Stick plant. He found tiny holes in the sheath below the attachment knot, holes through which body fluids from the vagina could escape into the sterile uterus if they wicked up the string. Crowder rejected the entire shipment—some 10 to 12 thousand Shields. He felt that the holes made the devices unsafe for use.

Charles Leys, one of Crowder's bosses at Chap Stick, sent a memo to Dave Mefford, A. H. Robins' quality control supervisor, asking for approval of the shipment of Shields Crowder had rejected.

"Attached are samples of Dalkon devices on which you will notice that the plastic sheath on the string has been stripped slightly or been mashed in tying," Leys wrote. "We have several thousand of these caused by the tightened knots sliding over that portion of the string. It seems that we will continually have this problem facing us and I will appreciate your examining these and letting us know if they are acceptable."

Crowder knew that his bosses at Chap Stick were trying to override his rejection of the shipment, and he decided he would have to prove to them the potential danger that the perforations in the sheath presented.

He conducted an experiment. He clipped several unknotted sections of strings from the shipment of Shields he had rejected, then stood the strings, which were semi-rigid, in beakers of water. Several hours later, he examined the strings under a microscope. Crowder was able to squeeze water from the "dry" ends of the string, the ends he had left out of the water. The strings definitely wicked.

But could water wick past the bottom knot on the string, the knot doctors used to make sure the device was positioned correctly in the uterus? Lerner said his experiments showed it couldn't, but Crowder decided to conduct an experiment of his own. He placed one end of knotted sections of the string—but not the knot itself—in a beaker of water for several days. When he returned he found that water could indeed be "milked" from the other end of the string. It had wicked right through the knot.

Crowder felt he now had the evidence he needed to convince his boss that the string was dangerous. He called Ross to his laboratory and demonstrated the string's wicking to him. Ross was anything but pleased. He angrily reminded Crowder that the string was not Crowder's responsibility and that he should leave it alone. Crowder told Ross that he could not, in good conscience, keep quiet about something that he felt could cause infection in the women who wore the Shield.

"Your conscience doesn't pay your salary," Crowder says Ross replied. Ross also told Crowder that he was being insubordinate by pursuing this matter; if he valued his job he would do as he was told and forget about the string.

A. H. Robins officials overruled Crowder's rejection of the shipment of Shields. "I don't believe the mashed thread that you referred to in your June 11 memo is a serious problem," Mefford wrote to Leys. (Copies of this memo went to the upper reaches of A. H. Robins—to E. C. Robins, Jr., who was soon to join the company's board of directors, and to Charles Morton, A. H. Robins' vice-president and general manager.) And so, some 10 to 12 thousand Shields, with strings containing microscopic holes in the sheaths, were shipped to doctors around the country and eventually found their way into the uteri of unsuspecting women.

While A. H. Robins apparently had no qualms about sending out Shields that were potentially dangerous to women, company executives continued to be very concerned about the "male sensitivity" problem. To soften the string, A. H. Robins instructed Chap Stick to boil the string before attempting to tie it. But this caused other problems. "Boiling too long can cause kinking and weakening," acknowledged one Chap Stick official in March. And Charles Leys wrote again to Mefford, in June 1971, to report that "the plastic sheet is more apt to strip off the line if it is boiled." Mefford, however, told Leys to keep boiling the string "because without thoroughly investigating the long-term benefits of boiling, I don't think we should incorporate a change."

By July, however, it was felt some change was needed. Crowder was called to Ross' office for a meeting with Daniel French, the president of Chap Stick. French wanted Crowder to compare the string stock currently being used at Chap Stick with earlier stock to see if the current stock was somehow stiffer—and thus more likely to be painful to men.

Crowder jumped on this opportunity to explain to French his concerns about the string. He described his wicking experiments and voiced his fear that water and bacteria traveling through the string could reach the sterile uterus and cause infection. French listened attentively. When Crowder was done, French said he agreed with his logic, that it sounded reasonable, and that he had heard some similar "scuttlebutt" in Richmond about infection and the Shield.

Encouraged, Crowder then demonstrated for French, as he had for Ross and Lerner, how the end of the string could be sealed by heat or flame. This beading, he said, might solve the problem of wicking and that of discomfort during intercourse reported by some men.

French said A. H. Robins would never go for the idea. He said the company had too much time and money invested in testing the present configuration of the device; if changes were made, all the tests would have to be redone. Also, heat sealing the end of the tail string would cost money.

Crowder tried to pursue his arguments, but French moved the discussion back to the problem of male sensitivity to the string. He told Crowder to begin his tests on the string's stiffness right away. "Maybe you can get some of the girls in the factory to help you with the testing," he joked.

After French left the meeting, Ross told Crowder that he hoped he had finally gotten the business about the string out of his system. Crowder, however, had no intention of leaving the problem alone. If neither Ross nor French would forward his concerns to A. H. Robins, he would do it himself.

On July 28, 1971, Crowder wrote up the results of his string stiffness tests in a memo to Ross. The tests had shown, he reported, that different reels of string did vary in stiffness and that boiling the string before tying would only produce a temporary softening effect.

But that wasn't the only topic of the memo. Because of the complexity of his tests, Crowder knew the memo would be forwarded to A. H. Robins officials. So he took the opportunity to go over his bosses' heads and make a direct pitch to A. H. Robins about his concerns over the string.

"I also question the value of the sheath (which contributes to the stiffness) since, as I understand its purpose, it is to keep the interior of the string dry and thus thwart bacterial growth," he wrote. "The string, however, has two exposed cut ends and, exposed to water can become wet inside. This can be demonstrated by immersing one end of the string to a beaker of water. After standing overnight, small droplets of water can be 'milked' out of the string end . . . Beading the end would eliminate the sharpness factor as well as sealing the string from wetting inside from capillary action."

Ross was furious when he received the memo. He called Crowder into his office and threatened again to fire him.

Whether the memo was ever sent to Richmond is unclear, but Crowder's basic concern about the string did make its way to Richmond via another route. On August 5, French called Ellen Preston at A. H. Robins to talk with her about the string. Chap Stick had noticed a couple of problems with the string, which he was sure the medical department would want to know about, he told her. After their conversation, Preston wrote a memo to Fred Clark.

"The string is very difficult to work with, and Mr. French suggested that alternate types of materials should be looked into," Preston wrote. "The sheath is a problem (I do not know exactly how) but I believe there is a problem with its stripping off if the cut ends are handled excessively. Mr. French says the reason given for the sheath is that it provides protection against bacterial invasion. He points out, however, that both ends of the string are cut and left open. It has been shown that the open ends will wick water. It seems to him if this is so then the ends will wick body fluids containing bacteria."

French was now passing on to A. H. Robins Crowder's warning to him. But the warning was again ignored. In fact, Clark called French and sharply rebuffed him for worrying about testing the Shield. Chap Stick should focus instead on getting the device assembled and packaged, Clark told him. French finally backed off. "As I indicated in our telephone conversation," he wrote back to Clark, "it is not the intention of the Chap Stick Company to attempt any unauthorized improvements in the Dalkon Shield. My only interest in the Dalkon Shield is to produce it at the lowest possible price and, therefore, increase Robins' gross profit level."

So Crowder was essentially silenced. He would, however, continue to reject shipments of Shields—and continue to be rebuffed for it. His future at Chap Stick grew dimmer and dimmer until eventually, during a company reorganization in 1978, he was "let go."

A. H. Robins officials say Crowder's study was dismissed because it wasn't scientific. "We hah-hahed [about] Crowder," recalls Jack Freund. "He wasn't medical, he was manufacturing."

A. H. Robins did not try to duplicate Crowder's wicking studies until 1974, after the Shield was taken off the market. Crowder's heat-sealing idea was also revived around that time—and then dismissed. "It is too late to 'heat seal' now," wrote Ellen Preston in a December 1974 memo to Fred Clark. "We need to *abandon* the 'multifilament' string. Heat-sealing would have been a good thing to have done 4 years ago."

However, as early as October 1971, A. H. Robins was frantically, albeit quietly, searching for an alternative tail string.

On October 11, 1971, yet another A. H. Robins official made the trip up to Stamford to talk with Lerner. This time it was Ken Moore, who had recently been appointed project manager for the Dalkon Shield. It was basically a "get-acquainted" meeting; much of the discussion centered on possible improvements in the Shield.

As his five-page memo of the meeting (which he sent to Roy Smith) showed, Moore was leery of Lerner. "Though I'm certain there is no one more interested in the continuing success of the Shield," Moore wrote, "there will be times when some controls will have to be placed upon him." Lerner, for his part, had expressed his displeasure with some A. H. Robins officials who he believed were giving both him and Davis the cold shoulder. Lerner and Davis were upset that Davis hadn't been consulted when A. H. Robins was devising its latest patient information sheet. They felt they should both be consulted on all advertising for the Shield.

Lerner also wanted to know who was going to be conducting future tests on experimental Shields—Lerner Laboratories or Chap Stick. Lerner said he preferred to keep his hand in on the testing, and Moore agreed with him. "If developmental work were left in Stamford, there would be less temptation for Chap Stick to make changes on their own," Moore wrote in his memo. A. H. Robins officials obviously had not been too pleased with the uproar over the tail string raised by Chap Stick a couple of months earlier.

But Moore didn't want Lerner running off and conducting tests on his own, either. "The main disadvantage to this approach [letting Lerner Laboratories stay in charge of developmental work on the Shield] is that this might encourage Lerner to conduct experimental studies without proper direction from Richmond in that he appears to be a rather independent man," Moore wrote. Lerner's independence was reflected in his response to Moore's suggestions for changes in the Shield's design. Lerner rejected most of them. Doctors, not the Shield's design, should be blamed, Lerner said, for any pain experienced by women during removal of the device. Lerner also expressed concern that changing the design now "could raise some questions as to whether or not we in fact know what we are doing."

Lerner, however, "was anxious to solve the string problem," Moore reported. Moore got a run-down from Lerner of the problems he had experienced testing various types of string. Monofilaments tore through the Shield itself and were difficult to tie. Braided strings supported bacterial growth. And even some coated braided strings (although naturally not one coated in nylon, as the Shield was) "most likely would support bacterial growth," Lerner told him.

Moore would spend the three years following his meeting with Lerner "desperately searching," as he later put it, for a new tail string.

One of the most perplexing problems of the tail string was the deterioration of its nylon sheath, usually several months after the Shield was inserted into a woman. This was particularly serious because, in theory at least, the nylon sheath was supposed to keep bacteria from entering the uterus. If the sheath deteriorated and microscopic holes formed in it, then bacteria could, and did, seep through.

Moore acknowledged the problem of deterioration in a February 1972 memo to Ellen Preston. "The possibility that the nylon is losing its integrity after several months in situ exists," he noted.

This concept shouldn't have been new to A. H. Robins officials. Studies as early as the 1950s had shown that nylon breaks down in water. In addition, the particular nylon used in the Dalkon Shield tail string— Nylon 6—was known to be hydrophilic, or water-attracting, making it even more likely to deteriorate. Other popular IUDs on the market during the early 1970s had strings made of materials that were water-repellent, making them less likely to wick.

In early 1972, Moore attended a meeting of a research committee involved with the Shield. "It was mentioned that studies have not been conducted to evaluate the effect of uterine and vaginal fluids on the string," he reported afterward. Yet no action was taken. The needed lab and animal tests were left undone.

A year later, Donald Ostergard, an obstetrician and gynecologist teaching at the University of California Medical School at Los Angeles who had already conducted a pregnancy study for A. H. Robins, asked the company to fund a study on bacteriological flora associated with the Dalkon Shield. Such a study could have determined whether the device caused infection. But A. H. Robins turned Ostergard down. "We just can't fit the price tag for this study into what we see as our needs for this shield over the next year or two," explained Ellen Preston.

But the problems with the string would not go away. Reports of pelvic infections caused by the Shield were arriving regularly at A. H. Robins' Richmond headquarters. On February 3, 1972, a doctor reported six cases of PID in approximately 290 insertions. In March, a very angry doctor from the University of Utah spoke with Gordon Brown of A. H. Robins' medical department. "[He] is very upset about the Dalkon Shield," Brown wrote in a memo about the conversation. "He said 5 girls in a row developed a pelvic infection; 3 of which had to be hospitalized. He said if he had his way it would be removed from the market."

The doctor was so angry, according to Brown, that, "it was impossible to discuss the problem with him." When Brown asked the doctor if he had inserted the Shield during the women's menstrual periods, the doctor shouted back, "I know what I'm doing. I've inserted more IUDs than you have." "I'm sure you have, doctor," Brown replied. "I haven't inserted any."

A month later, a professor at the Medical University of South Carolina reported two more cases of Dalkon Shield-related PID to A. H. Robins, including another case of a woman who became so ill that she had to be hospitalized.

In April 1972, A. H. Robins hired John Autian, an expert plastics toxicologist from the University of Tennessee, to come to Richmond and consult on whether EVA, the plastic used in the Shield, was toxic. Autian made several suggestions on the kinds of tests A. H. Robins should conduct to determine the short- and long-range effects of the device on the bodies of the women wearing it. Autian told Moore that he didn't believe EVA would prove to be a problem.

The nylon string, however, was another story. "[Autian] feels we have a definite problem with [the nylon string] because historically it has been shown that nylon does deteriorate in situ over a period of time," Moore noted in a memo of their meeting that went to Jack Freund and Roy Smith. Autian recommended that A. H. Robins conduct tests on the nylon string as well as on the plastic in the body of the device, and he recommended alternate materials—Dacron, polyethylene, and polypropylene—for the string.

Soon after Autian's visit, Moore wrote another memo, this one handwritten and addressed to Ellen Preston. "As you know, we are desperately searching for a suitable material to replace our currently used nylon string. We hope to locate something no later than June 1. We have some good leads at this time." Moore wanted a monofilament, not a multifilament string. "Our end goal at this point is to find a suitable polyester monofilament to be used as the Dalkon Shield tail," he said in yet another memo.

The June deadline was not met, however. By the fall of 1972, Moore was still searching for a new string. It had to be soft and flexible, yet strong enough to withstand the stress of tugging during removal and of twisting during tying. And, it could not wick or deteriorate in situ. Moore made that clear in his correspondence with string manufacturers.

In November, Moore felt he had found the string he wanted in a material with the brand name Gore-Tex. But the new string was never used. Just why it was rejected is unclear. It may have had something to do with cost. The new string would have cost A. H. Robins six cents more per Shield—or 10 times the cost of the Supramid they were already using. A. H. Robins officials insist this wasn't the reason the Gore-Tex string was rejected. They say the new string was rejected because it was too weak and too slippery. (Doctors would have had the inconvenience of using special instruments to grab hold of the slippery string during removal. Perhaps A. H. Robins was worried this inconvenience would turn doctors away from the Shield.)

But there was yet another reason. The Gore-Tex string was too stiff. It didn't solve the "male sensitivity" problem.

So despite warnings that the Shield string could deteriorate and allow bacteria to get into a woman's uterus, causing potentially life-threatening infections; and despite reports from doctors that this was indeed occurring, A. H. Robins stayed with the original string. The Gore-Tex alternative was abandoned because, in addition to costing more, it would still—as a Minnesota attorney later crudely put it—"prick men's pricks."

What it could do to the health of women seemed to be of little concern.

Peggy

"We're lucky to have Melissa. Very lucky."
—Peggy McClean Mample, October 1984.

On July 5, 1971, just one month after graduating from Borah High School in Boise, Idaho, Peggy McClean married her high school sweetheart, John Bown, a dashing black-haired, blue-eyed young man who had recently enlisted in the Navy. It was the storybook wedding that many high school girls dream about—the bride in a long white gown, the groom in a white tuxedo, and the service in a charming clapboard church with a tall white steeple.

Like all young couples, Peggy and John had a vision of their life together. He wanted to become a football coach; she wanted to put her enthusiasm for dance and sports into a career as a physical education teacher.

Both also wanted to have children—although not right away. Peggy had started taking birth control pills about a month before their marriage.

Within days of their wedding, Peggy and John left Idaho for the Whidbey Island Naval Air Station in western Washington, where John had been ordered to report for duty. They moved into a tiny trailer near the base.

During the move, Peggy lost her prescription for her birth control pills, so she went to the Navy infirmary and got a second, different prescription. These new pills created problems for Peggy. They affected her moods, making her very emotional at times, and they caused her to put on weight. Peggy returned to the infirmary and was given a different type of pill, but the unwanted mood-swings and weight-gain persisted. On her third trip to the infirmary, she asked if there was something else she could take or use for contraception that would be as effective as the Pill, but less troublesome.

Her doctor recommended an IUD—specifically, the Dalkon Shield IUD. He told her it was as safe and effective as the Pill. Two months later, during her menstrual period, Peggy returned to have a Dalkon Shield inserted. As her doctor had warned, the insertion was slightly painful, but it was soon over and Peggy went home, glad she was off the Pill.

But Peggy soon discovered that she had traded one set of problems for another. After the Shield was inserted, her periods became very heavy and painful. She found that while menstruating she had to take frequent breaks from her job as a clerk at a local five-and-dime store. When she wasn't resting, she would be in the bathroom changing her menstrual pad as frequently as every hour.

In January 1972, three months after the Shield was inserted, Peggy did not menstruate at all. She suspected immediately that she was pregnant and called the base infirmary, but was told to wait until she had missed a second period before coming in for a pregnancy test.

The wait was hard and Peggy became increasingly distraught as she thought about being pregnant. She didn't want to be pregnant. She and John could not afford a baby. But even more important, Peggy did not want to give up her new-found independence. She enjoyed being away from Boise and her family, enjoyed being essentially on her own. But as the wait continued, Peggy began to think more and more about the baby that might be within her womb until one day she knew she could never abort it. She was going to have that baby, and, she told herself, it was going to be a little girl.

The pregnancy was confirmed in March. Peggy's doctor explained that a decision had to be made about the Shield. The Shield could be left inside her uterus for the entire pregnancy, or it could be removed. In either case, she would have a 50 percent chance of miscarrying the baby. The act of removing the device could trigger a miscarriage; if left in, the device could cause a miscarriage by making the uterus contract. Peggy decided to keep the Shield in.

The first few months of the pregnancy went well. Peggy kept physically active, but she curtailed her dancing. At night, as she felt the baby move within her, Peggy sometimes would dream of how she would teach the child to dance, of how they might even dance together on stage one day.

Early in July, Peggy began to experience severe cramps—similar to the cramps she had experienced after the IUD was inserted. She was very concerned, for she was only six months pregnant. She spoke to her doctor about the cramps, but he told her not to worry, that it was probably only false labor. He told her it was not necessary to come in for a special checkup. *He thinks I'm just another neurotic pregnant woman,* Peggy thought to herself.

On July 20, almost two weeks after the cramps had begun, Peggy went in for her regularly-scheduled seven-month checkup. After giving Peggy a pelvic exam, the doctor remained unconcerned about the cramps. He did, however, give her a prescription for what he believed might be a urinary tract infection. Peggy had been urinating frequently in recent weeks—too frequently, the doctor believed. (The results of a urine test taken that day later showed she had no infection.)

Peggy had the prescription filled, then went home. That night, while standing at the sink making ice tea for her husband, she felt a rush of water from her vagina. It spilled out from under her dress and made a puddle on the kitchen floor. Peggy thought that the pills the doctor had given her had made her lose control of her bladder and urinate. She cleaned up the mess, then laid down on her living room couch. Each time she moved, more liquid would seep from between her legs.

All through the night the cramps grew in intensity, shooting through her abdomen at regular intervals. In the morning, Peggy went into the bathroom to urinate and it was then that she discharged a plug of greyish mucus laced with blood. This was the "show," a sign that labor has begun. Peggy was terrified. It was too early. She was only seven months pregnant.

John called the naval hospital and was told to bring Peggy in right away. At the hospital, a doctor quickly confirmed that she was in labor and pulled out her Dalkon Shield, which had slipped down into her cervical canal. Peggy heard the "clink" as the doctor dropped it into a metal waste can.

Things then began to happen very fast. Because the naval hospital was not equipped to care for premature babies, Peggy was rushed by helicopter to the University of Washington Hospital 90 miles away. During the ride, the pilot and a Navy physician talked to Peggy and kept her spirits up. An ambulance was waiting when the helicopter touched down, and Peggy was whisked to the University Hospital. From then on, everything was a blur for Peggy. She remembers people with solemn faces and somber voices walking in and out of the labor room. She remembers the *pain of hard labor and begging the anesthesiologist for pain medicine right before delivery. But most of all, she remembers being terrified for her baby, who was being born two months prematurely.*

At 1:46 A.M. on Saturday, July 22, 1972, some 27 hours after she first went into labor, Peggy gave birth to a three-pound, five-ounce baby girl with dark hair whom she named Melissa. Although the child had arrived sooner than she had expected, Peggy had the little girl she wanted, the little girl she hoped one day to teach to dance.

But from the start, Melissa had problems. She was born with a hyaline membrane disease, sometimes called infant respiratory distress syndrome (IRDS), a disease that afflicts some 25,000 newborn babies each year. Because Melissa's lungs were not fully developed, they lacked "pulmonary surfactant," a substance that normally reduces the "stickiness" within the lung's air sacs, enabling the lungs to expand. Melissa had to struggle for every breath.

Melissa also had jaundice and dislocated hips. But, by far, the biggest concern was the hyaline membrane disease. At the time, 30 to 50 percent of babies born with the disease died. Ten years earlier, one of those babies had been John and Jacqueline Kennedy's infant son, Patrick.

Melissa was in an isolette for a month. When visiting her, Peggy and John had to scrub their hands and forearms for five minutes, then put on hospital caps, gowns, and gloves. Even then they could only touch her through the protective holes of the isolette. The nurses taught Peggy and John how to tap the isolette if Melissa stopped breathing to stimulate her into breathing again. Several times during their visits, Melissa did stop breathing and her terrified parents would tap and tap until she started again.

Melissa's lungs gradually recovered, until she was able to breathe regularly and strongly on her own. When she was about four weeks old and out of immediate danger, she was transferred to the Whidbey Island Naval Hospital where doctors said she would have to remain until she weighed at least five pounds. Melissa reached that magical weight on September 5, when she was about six weeks old. Peggy and John proudly carried their still-tiny daughter home.

Soon after Melissa came home, John was transferred back to Boise. Peggy did not get another job outside the home, preferring instead to spend her days and nights taking care of Melissa. And Melissa needed a lot of care. Because of her dislocated hips, she had to be "double-diapered," that is, a diaper was wrapped around each leg to keep her legs splayed apart. When she was a few months old, she was big enough to fit into a small U-shaped brace that had the same effect. She remained in that brace for a year.

Peggy was always watching Melissa for signs of brain damage. The lack of oxygen that occurs with hyaline membrane disease can cause small brain hemorrhages, which, in turn, can leave damaging scar tissue inside the brain.

For the first few months, Peggy saw no evidence that Melissa was falling behind in her development. Melissa did not sit up at six months, but Peggy just attributed it to the fact that Melissa was actually only four months old and therefore should not be expected to sit up. At nine months, however, Melissa was still not sitting up. She had to be propped into a sitting position, and even then it seemed an unnatural position for her. Her hips were too stiff; they didn't bend easily. Nor did Melissa move around in the natural way. Instead of crawling on hands and knees, Melissa scooted around on her back, eventually rubbing a temporary bald spot on the back of her head where it met the floor.

Peggy could tell that Melissa's pediatrician was concerned. He began to prepare Peggy for the possibility that Melissa had suffered some brain damage during her premature birth. When Melissa was 13 months old, he suggested they take some tests, including an EEG of Melissa's brain.

The resulting diagnosis was clear—Melissa had spastic diplegia, a form of cerebral palsy. Although she had expected the diagnosis, Peggy was still devastated when she heard it. She could not bring herself to tell her husband at first, who for months had refused to believe anything was wrong with Melissa. Even after he was told, John refused to accept it. Gradually, he withdrew—from Melissa, from Peggy, from the marriage.

Peggy, however, decided to tackle Melissa's illness head-on. She immediately enrolled Melissa in physical therapy classes, and then insisted on learning how to do the therapy herself with Melissa at home. Night after night, she would work with Melissa, gently pulling and twisting her legs and arms to increase her daughter's flexibility.

Their first goal was to get Melissa to sit up on her own. That day came when Melissa was 18 months old. Peggy cried with joy as she watched her daughter pull herself into a sitting position and then stay seated. By the time she was two years old, Melissa could walk short distances with the aid of leg braces and a walker. She was also talking quite well. Much to Peggy's relief, the damage experienced by Melissa at birth had not affected her mental abilities.

Melissa grew into a beautiful child, with big blue eyes and straight brown hair. When she was two years old, and again when she was three, *she was chosen by the Idaho chapter of the March of Dimes to be its poster child. Wearing her braces and a broad smile, she was photographed often with Idaho politicians during those years.*

But not everything was going well for Peggy. Her marriage with John was falling apart, in large part because he could just not accept his daughter's handicaps. Peggy became pregnant again, thinking a second, healthy child might save the marriage; but it didn't, and in December 1974 she found herself divorced with custody of a handicapped two-year-old and a six-month-old baby boy.

It was a very difficult time for Peggy. She moved in with her sister and began working at Kentucky Fried Chicken, a job that paid only $2.50 an hour and came with no medical benefits. Peggy didn't know how she would pay Melissa's bills, which were mounting daily. Melissa had developed what doctors call inflammatory asthma, and each cold or case of the flu that Melissa contracted developed into asthma. Peggy repeatedly had to rush her to the hospital, often in the middle of the night, for a shot of epinephrine.

There were other health problems as well. One day, while Peggy was in the kitchen, she heard a strange noise from the living room. She ran into the other room and saw Melissa shaking uncontrollably on the floor; blood from her nose was running down her face. Melissa was having a seizure, one of several she would experience during the next few years.

Peggy quit her job and went on welfare. It was the only way she knew of to take care of her daughter's medical needs. She had investigated joining the Navy, but she had no one to look after her children for the nine weeks of boot camp.

When Melissa was two, she had two operations on her hips. Doctors hoped the surgery would give her more normal hip movement, that it might even enable her to walk, if only haltingly. But when Melissa was six, it became clear that even with the surgery, she would never be able to walk more than the very shortest of distances. Her doctors recommended a wheelchair.

The wheelchair arrived on a warm May morning, and Peggy watched Melissa sit in it for the first time. As she watched, Peggy finally let go of the dream she had been carrying with her since before Melissa's birth. She realized her daughter would never dance. Nor would she enjoy the other activities that Peggy had loved so much as a child—playing the piano or baseball, riding a bicycle, climbing trees. She would be confined to her wheelchair, or to dragging herself along on the floor, her legs trailing her like heavy, dead weights.

The year was 1976. The Dalkon Shield had been off the market for two years and doctors had now been warned to remove the Shield from women who became pregnant while wearing it. Peggy had always suspected that the Shield had something to do with Melissa's premature birth, although doctors had always been vague when she brought it up.

Years later, Peggy would learn the truth about Melissa's birth. After seven months of pregnancy, at the time when the womb becomes sensitive and begins to contract, Peggy's uterus had developed an inflammatory reaction to the Shield. This reaction had triggered labor and led to Melissa's premature birth, the hyaline membrane disease, and, ultimately, the cerebral palsy.

In September 1982, Peggy filed a lawsuit against A. H. Robins.

"The more I read, the more I understood," she explains. "The [A. H. Robins Company] was just raping all the American women, women all over the world . . . I will probably always be angry."

10

Counterattack

"Before 1970, IUDs were seldom considered as a contraceptive method of first choice. The Dalkon Shield is changing that."
—Dalkon Shield "Progress Report,"
advertisement to physicians, November 1972.

By mid-1972, more and more doctors were discovering that the Dalkon Shield was not as free of complications as Hugh Davis and A. H. Robins would have them believe. In fact, the Shield was developing a growing reputation among medical professionals for having a high pregnancy rate, for being difficult to insert and remove, and for causing infections.

One of the first indications that doctors were bad-mouthing the Shield came in March 1972 when A. H. Robins officials learned that Dr. H. Oliver Williamson, a South Carolina doctor, had spoken disparagingly about the device to a group of general practitioners. The doctor had quoted Dr. Howard Tatum, a well-known population and IUD expert, as saying, "You know the Dalkon Shield is no good, I know it's no good, but there is no documentation to this effect in the literature."

A tape of the doctor's comments to the general practitioners was recorded without the doctor's knowledge and made its way to Richmond, where it caused quite a stir and a flurry of memos. Ellen Preston wrote to the doctor to tell him that "reports to us (even scanty ones) of pelvic infection associated with the Shield have been very rare—particularly when the extensive use of this device is considered." The doctor was not so easily reassured. A few days after receiving the letter from Preston, he sent A. H. Robins a report of a patient who had "developed a severe

96

inflammatory process involving the uterus, ovaries, Fallopian tubes, and parametrial tissue in association with the Dalkon Shield."

On June 23, 1972, Thad Earl wrote to Richmond to tell John Burke, A. H. Robins' general sales manager, that he had heard complaints about the Shield in discussions with doctors at two recent medical conventions.

In the letter Earl wondered "if money and politics are involved because when I try to nail down these people the investigators and cases seem to vanish." Yet, in that same letter Earl acknowledged that he was intimately aware of at least several problem cases because he had seen them firsthand—they involved his own patients. These new cases indicated that the Shield could cause a rare and extremely serious health threat to women—spontaneous septic abortions, or miscarriages accompanied by infections. Despite the significance of these cases, Earl didn't mention them until page three of his five-page letter, and then only as part of a discussion on how he was countering complaints from doctors.

"The next situation I have found is with women becoming pregnant and if the Shield is left in place the women abort at 3½ to 5 months and become septic. I am advising physicians that the device should be removed as soon as a diagnosis of pregnancy is made. Numerous physicians have noted this. In my six pregnancies, I removed one and she carried full term, the rest all aborted and became septic. I therefore feel it is hazardous to leave the device in and I advised that it be removed. I realize that this is a small statistic but I feel we should correlate this data with other investigators across the country, because most men are experiencing the same problem."

Earl ended the letter by telling Burke that he was moving to Lordsburg, New Mexico, within a few days. (Earl had been hospitalized in the fall of 1971 and was told by a cardiologist to either cut back or quit his practice.) He gave Burke his new address.

A. H. Robins had now been put on notice by one of its own consultants that the Shield might be causing septic abortions. Yet company officials made no effort at that time to look into the matter. In fact, they didn't even respond to Earl's letter until three months later.

"I was most interested in your suggestion that the Dalkon Shield be removed when a diagnosis of pregnancy is made," Ken Moore, the Shield's project manager, wrote to Earl on August 22, 1972. "This is completely in reverse of what we have been recommending since it was felt that the pregnancy would have a better chance of continuing to term if the Dalkon Shield were left in place. Any documentation of cases reported to you would be considerably helpful in our establishing an official position on this very important aspect. Hopefully, our clinical data summary will shed some light on this also." (The company was conducting a survey of doctors regarding their clinical use of the Shield.)

Earl says he never received the letter from Moore, and, thus, didn't respond to Moore's request for more information. And Moore never pursued Earl any further to get the documentation he asked for.

Only after two years—and reports of several women dying from septic abortions—would A. H. Robins do what Earl had recommended and put out a general warning to doctors to remove the Shield from women who become pregnant while wearing it.

Although some doctors may have been learning the truth about problems with the Shield, the word was much slower in reaching the women who wore or were considering wearing the device. Part of the reason for this delay was an extensive promotional campaign A. H. Robins launched in late 1971, a campaign aimed directly at women.

Drug companies don't usually advertise their prescription products directly to consumers, because it usually does not make economic sense to do so. Doctors, after all, make most prescription choices for their patients. But the Dalkon Shield was different. Through its market research A. H. Robins had discovered that many women asked specifically for a particular brand of IUD. Naturally, A. H. Robins wanted that brand to be the Dalkon Shield. So the company decided to make their pitch to women as well as doctors.

In October 1971, Bob Nickless wrote to Hugh Davis to tell him that he would soon be contacted by Richard Wilcox, a public relations man from New York City "who has been retained to get some lay publicity for us on the Dalkon Shield." A. H. Robins had recently contracted with Wilcox's firm, Wilcox and Williams, for $2,500 a month (plus expenses) to get favorable coverage in the popular press for the Dalkon Shield. E. Claiborne Robins, Sr., had himself assigned "top priority" to this "special promotion of the Dalkon Shield in other than medical and trade magazines," as Richard Velz, A. H. Robins' own public relations man, and the person considered to be E. Claiborne's "right hand man" in the company, reported in a memo.

Wilcox's assignment was to plant articles favorable to the Shield in general circulation magazines. He did his job well. Editors were very receptive to stories about the Shield. In January 1972, for example, Wilcox arranged a meeting between a doctor from A. H. Robins' medical department and an editor from *Mademoiselle* magazine. "This visit has resulted in the assignment of an article by the editor, Mary Cantwell, to a writer," reported Wilcox in a progress report to Robins officials. "The article will be on contraception in general, with emphasis on the Dalkon Shield. Mary Cantwell states that her decision was based on Dr. Chremos' [from A. H. Robins] visit and his excellent presentation to her staff of the subject in general and the Dalkon Shield in particular." Dr. Chremos also met with the editor of *Family Circle* to add information for an article the editor had already contracted from Davis.

In mid-February, Wilcox arranged for Nickless to meet with a reporter from the Kyodo News Service, a wire service used by all newspapers in Japan and many in other countries around the world. "This meeting and subsequent back-up material resulted in an article favorable to the Dalkon Shield . . . for distribution to Kyodo's full list," reported Wilcox. "In addition, the material on the Dalkon Shield was forwarded to Kyodo's Economic News Bureau, which services banks, brokerage houses, insurance companies and other industrial and commercial customers."

Wilcox also noted in his progress report that syndicated columnist Barbara Seaman wrote two articles that favorably mentioned the Dalkon Shield that were carried by the *Baltimore Sun*, the *Kansas City Star*, and some 40 other newspapers. According to Wilcox, Seaman also planned to refer favorably to the Shield in her book, *Free and Female*, which was scheduled to be published that spring.

More than 10 years later, Seaman, a well-known feminist and medical writer, says she does not recall being contacted by Wilcox or anyone from A. H. Robins about the Dalkon Shield. She says it is possible she mentioned the Shield in her syndicated column "out of a courtesy" to Hugh Davis, who had written a foreword to her 1969 book *The Doctors' Case Against the Pill*. Seaman does recall being asked later by Davis to write an article favorable to the Shield for *Family Circle* magazine, but she says she decided against it. She had by then developed serious reservations about the safety of IUDs.

Wilcox had successfully nudged other references to the Shield—all favorable, of course—into print. One of his biggest successes was a column called "Health Highlights," which was produced as a kind of news release by Wilcox and Williams and printed verbatim in dozens of small newspapers throughout the country. It was a thinly disguised promo for IUDs in general—and the Dalkon Shield in particular.

"When it comes to family planning, three million American women can't be wrong! That is the number of American females who have chosen to use the intra-uterine device (IUD) to avert the birth of unwanted children," declared the column's lead paragraph. The column then went on to proclaim the advantages of the IUD over the Pill—and the specific advantages of the Dalkon Shield, "a new IUD which has been successfully used even in women who have never been pregnant."

But then the column took a wrong turn. "A report from Johns Hopkins University details trials with this Shield on more than five thousand women," the article reported. "Of this overall group, only one percent became pregnant." The column was wrong. Five thousand women had not been inserted with Dalkon Shields in "trials" at Johns Hopkins. What the column was undoubtedly referring to was Davis' mention in his *American Journal of Obstetrics & Gynecology* article of 5,000 women who had been fitted at John Hopkins with a variety of IUDs, not just the Dalkon Shield. With the Shield, Davis had only documented 640 insertions.

The column appeared in newspapers well into 1973, when Roger Tuttle, the A. H. Robins attorney responsible for the labeling of the Shield, found out about it and became furious. He thought the entire lay promotion campaign was highly unethical and ordered it stopped immediately. But on January 10, 1974, Tuttle received a memo from John Taylor of A. H. Robins' public relations office, "I talked with Dick Wilcox about the IUD column that highlighted the Dalkon Shield," Taylor reported. "The mechanics of recalling such a column are difficult and could lead to questioning and problems." Consequently, the company decided to let the column—and the grossly inaccurate information it was carrying—"expire quietly."

In the meantime, thousands of women were getting the message that the Dalkon Shield was a superior choice of birth control. And it was influencing their choices at doctors' offices. As Ken Moore noted in a company memo, there was a jump in sales from 12 percent of ob-gyns using the Shield in 1971 to 33 percent prescribing it in 1972, a jump he attributed to the company's lay promotion. "It appears that we are beginning to reap some benefits from Dick Wilcox's efforts," Moore wrote.

It wasn't only through the popular press that A. H. Robins was reaching women. The company also distributed thousands of patient information sheets and brochures to doctors, who were asked to put them in their waiting rooms for women to read. (Ironically, years later another set of brochures about the Dalkon Shield would also find their way into doctors' waiting rooms, brochures written by attorneys looking for Dalkon Shield victims to represent.)

These materials, targeted to patients, contained some extraordinary statements. One patient information sheet even claimed that women would have a better chance of reaching an orgasm with the Shield. "A recent survey of women using the Dalkon Shield noted a marked improvement in sexual relations," noted the patient information sheet. "Some of them found it much easier to reach an orgasm than with the other methods of contraception. This is another reason why wearing a Dalkon Shield can be a rewarding experience in your married life." (An A. H. Robins official says the "survey" was an informal one, conducted by Davis at Johns Hopkins during his discussion with his patients as he examined them.)

Many of the statements found in the patient brochures are highly misleading. They don't tell the full story behind the Shield and other IUDs. For example, the Shield's two November 1971 patient information sheets make the following statements:

- "IUDs are being used by millions of women throughout the world and have demonstrated outstanding medical safety." No mention was made of PID or perforations or of difficult removals resulting in operations.
- "The pregnancy rates with the modern pills and the modern Dalkon Shield IUD are similar." No mention was made of Davis' extended study which showed the Dalkon Shield's pregnancy rate was not comparable with that of the Pill.
- "Some women have cramps caused by insertion. These usually pass away in a few minutes, but may last longer." No mention was made of complaints from doctors and women about difficult and excruciatingly painful insertions, and that the women for whom cramps lasted "longer" suffered weeks and even months of pain.
- "There is a special threadlike tail on the Shield which projects through the mouth of the womb . . . It will not bother you or your husband during relations." No mention was made of A. H. Robins' internal dilemma over the "male sensitivity" problem and its attempt to soften the string through boiling.
- "Removal of the Shield restores your natural fertility and conception is once again possible. Most women who wish to become pregnant do so within three to six months after the IUD is removed." This was perhaps the most bitterly ironic statement in the brochure. The fact that "most women" who wished it became pregnant after removal of the Shield is little consolation to thousands of women who claim they were never able to have children as a result of infections caused by the Shield.

Despite A. H. Robins' promotional efforts, however, Dalkon Shield sales began to slump around mid-1972. A. H. Robins blamed the slump on "unsubstantiated 'pot shots' " from doctors and others—including a statement by the insurance manager at Planned Parenthood's national headquarters that 50 percent of the IUD perforations reported to Planned Parenthood clinics involved the Dalkon Shield. A. H. Robins also blamed the Shield's faltering image on "a minority but vociferous group of physicians" who had failed to insert the Shield correctly and were now trying to put the blame on the device rather than on their own "ignorance" or "indifference." They also blamed the sales slump on "the company's failure to get the 'good word' out about the Dalkon Shield"; the "lack of physician support for the Dalkon Shield at the major fertility meetings"; and the company's "failure to establish a good and lasting rapport with important family planning and population control groups around the country and the world." In other words, the bad reports about the Shield were a result of poor public relations, not poor design.

A. H. Robins officials decided a new and bold offensive was needed to shore up support for the Shield. In November 1972, A. H. Robins began its second advertising blitz aimed at doctors. Its cornerstone was an eight-page color advertisement, which the company dubbed a "progress report," and which ran in major obstetrical and gynecological journals. It is believed to be the biggest advertisement ever produced for an IUD.

The advertisement is interesting for several reasons, not the least of which is the patronizing way it treats women. Above photographs of worried-looking women, the ad asks the question, "Who are candidates for the Dalkon Shield?" then answers it this way:

"The applications of the Dalkon Shield are so universal that they cut across all socio-economic lines. They include all women who are not sufficiently motivated to take the Pill, ranging from the clinic patient to the busy mother-career woman who has so many activities and interests that taking a pill simply slips her mind. They also include your patient who is so disorganized she can't seem to get anything done on schedule." The message was clear—women cannot be trusted with birth control. They either lacked the motivation, or were too absent-minded or too disorganized to be in charge of their own fertility.

The ad also reiterates the claims A. H. Robins had made in its earlier promotion of the device: The Shield is a "superior contraception," with better retention and greater comfort than other IUDs and offers an improved method of insertion. To back up these claims, A. H. Robins printed the results of four published clinical studies in the ad. These studies, the ad said, "substantiate the low pregnancy and expulsion rates of the Dalkon Shield. In 3,174 insertions and after 17,222 woman-months of use . . . the pregnancy rate ranged from .5% to 1.9% and the expulsion rate from .2% to 2.3%. Note that there were 1,276 nulliparous patients in the four studies."

The first of these studies was Davis' 12-month study of 640 women. A. H. Robins did not change Davis' 1.1 percent pregnancy rate, although it knew it to be false. Nor did the ad acknowledge that Davis received royalties from Shield sales and was a paid consultant to the company.

The second study was Earl's 15-month study of 536 women, which had been prepared with A. H. Robins' assistance. Again, the company did not mention its role in the production of the study, nor did A. H. Robins note Earl's consulting contract with them or the royalties he was receiving on Shield sales. Nor did the company report Earl's warning about removing the Shield from women who became pregnant while wearing it to avoid dangerous septic abortions.

The third study cited in the progress report ad was one by Donald Ostergard. At A. H. Robins' request, he had begun a study on the Dalkon Shield at the Los Angeles County Harbor General Hospital. The study had been published in the November 1971 issue of *Contraception*.

Like Davis, Ostergard reported a 1.1 pregnancy rate, but a much higher medical removal rate (devices removed for pain or bleeding)—9.7 percent compared to Davis' reported two percent. But what A. H. Robins didn't note in the ad was that Ostergard's testing protocol had been severely criticized by the company's own biostatistician some nine months before the progress report ran.

Ostergard was one of 10 investigators selected by A. H. Robins to take part in a series of prospective Shield studies for the company. The first investigator had been recruited in December 1970, one month before the company began its original promotional blitz for the Shield; Ostergard joined the team nine months later, in August 1971.

The 10 studies, which collectively became known as the "Ten Investigator Prospective Study," were intended to follow some 2,000 Dalkon Shield wearers for at least two years. Although preliminary findings were used by A. H. Robins in 1973 to make changes in the Dalkon Shield's labeling, the study's final results (compiled in 1975) were never published by A. H. Robins—"and will not be published," according to Fletcher Owen, of Robins' medical staff. "There's some inconsistencies in the conduct of the study at the different centers," Owen said in 1985. ". . . I would say that the studies were not conclusive." Yet for years, Owen and other A. H. Robins officials publicly touted the Ten Investigator Prospective Study as the "Cadillac of the IUD studies." But not privately, within the company. On February 4, 1972, A. H. Robins' biostatistician, Lester

Preston (who was also Ellen Preston's husband), wrote an angry memo to Fred Clark in A. H. Robins' medical department (with a copy to Jack Freund) damning the data Ostergard had collected to that date for the Ten Investigator Prospective Study. Preston called for a suspension of all further use of data generated by the California doctor.

"I find it difficult, without producing a compendium, to say exactly what the problems are that we all seem to be facing [with Ostergard's work]," Preston wrote, "but they include such facts as multiple data sheets—not agreeing in content, from the same patients; many, many obvious 'errors' in completing the forms (i.e. obvious inconsistencies)—as well as ambiguities; gross deviations from protocol instructions (a la Tieze) with respect to such things as 'Lost to Follow-up' and 'Release From Follow-up'; questionable patient selection; administrative aspects (e.g. designating re-insertion patients as a new patient); etc. Our experience with the retrospective data that we have handled indicates that it, too, is flagrantly different and fraught with the *most obvious* errors."

Preston went on to call Ostergard's *Contraception* article (the one referred to in the progress report ad) "sloppy to say the least" and said that Ellen Preston agreed with him on that. "Frankly, my biggest fear is that we . . . can only see the 'tip-of-the-iceberg,'" Preston added. "I dislike the expression, but this could well turn out to be a clear-cut case of GIGO." (GIGO is a computer term for "garbage-in, garbage-out.") "As you well know, we expect 'problems' with all clinical data," Preston concluded, "but, as compared to other Dalkon Shield investigators, Dr. Ostergard's has created an essentially intolerable situation."

Twelve years later, Freund would smile when asked about Preston's memo and claim the statistician was obsessed with perfection and was just being picky in his evaluation of Ostergard. But in 1972, A. H. Robins officials ignored Preston's strong warnings about Ostergard's data and went ahead and used it in its progress report ad and in the packet of materials it sent out to physicians who wrote in with complaints.

The fourth study A. H. Robins used in its progress report advertisement was one published by Dr. Mary Gabrielson in an April 1972 issue of *Advances in Planned Parenthood*. In that article Gabrielson reported on her preliminary data from a study conducted on women at two California Planned Parenthood clinics. This preliminary data, gathered after nine months, reflected a favorable 1.9 percent pregnancy rate for the Dalkon Shield (but a high medical removal rate of 14.9 percent).

However, in April 1972, some seven months before the progress report ad ran, Gabrielson revised her data after allowing for a longer follow-up period of 14 months. She now reported a much higher pregnancy rate of

4.3 percent (and a much higher medical removal rate as well—24.4 percent). Gabrielson presented her more complete and accurate results to a conference of the American Association of Planned Parenthood Physicians in Detroit on April 6, 1972. Ken Moore was there and later wrote a memo which was sent to a long list of A. H. Robins officials. They were also notified of Gabrielson's higher pregnancy findings in a letter from Ostergard.

The final results of Gabrielson's study were published in the May 1972 issue of *Family Planning Digest*, an official publication of the Department of Health, Education and Welfare. By then the findings reflected 18 months of data. Gabrielson now reported a 5.1 percent pregnancy rate and a 26.4 percent medical removal rate. She also reported a 5 percent infection rate and warned doctors that "when pain is encountered with the IUD, the clinician should carefully consider the possibility of infection . . . but it may be caused by endometritis, parametritis, or salpingitis—all of which need immediate attention." (Despite these numbers, Gabrielson still considered the Shield an acceptable form of contraception.)

A. H. Robins ignored Gabrielson's final findings, preferring instead to publish her more favorable nine-month results in its progress ad and other promotional materials.

So the four studies boldly presented to doctors as evidence of the Shield's effectiveness and safety included two studies by doctors with a financial interest in the Shield; one study whose findings were seriously questioned by a member of A. H. Robins' own staff; and a study that, in its final form, had come to a less favorable conclusion about the Shield than the ad professed.

Besides running the progress report ad, A. H. Robins officials decided to hire seven ob-gyns as consultants, doctors who were "experienced and successful Dalkon Shield users" who could troubleshoot for the company against the Shield's detractors. The company also decided to seek out favorable data about the Dalkon Shield. In January 1973, Ken Moore sent a memo to Ellen Preston about a Dr. Dominguez who had written a paper on another IUD. "It might not be a bad idea to touch base with Dr. Dominguez," Moore advised Preston, "to see what his current experiences are with the Dalkon Shield, and if favorable, to determine if he would be interested in participating in a retrospective study."

That same month Moore wrote another memo to Preston with the same theme. He told Preston that "considering some of the adverse comments [about problems with the Shield] coming out of Planned Parenthood centers around the country, and particularly National Headquarters, I think it is most important that we encourage in every way possible Dr. Moorhead [a Planned Parenthood doctor in Columbus, Ohio] to present and/or publish favorable Dalkon Shield data." Preston phoned Moorhead, a call she noted in a memo to her files: "I told Dr. Moorhead, as I had before that we would pay $2.00 or so per case record to obtain the Dalkon Shield data from this clinic or perhaps even somewhat more. We obviously are not interested in paying premium prices for unfavorable data, but that his data, at least his estimate of it, was favorable."

Another letter with the same theme was sent to researchers at Providence Lying-In Hospital in Massachusetts. "As I indicated to you during our telephone conversation," Preston wrote to the researchers, "I am not very amenable at this point to expending a great deal of money or personnel time to analyze Dalkon Shield data which is anticipated to be unfavorable."

It is clear that A. H. Robins was interested only in getting favorable, rather than complete, data about the Shield. But favorable data about the Shield was hard to come by, as Preston admits in a report dated August 1973.

"We have, prior to the maturity of our own studies, attempted to pick up some quick, favorable statistics by retrospectively analyzing data made available to us," Preston wrote. "Most attempts at this have failed in that anticipated low (around 2%) pregnancy rates have been higher. To date, none of these studies have been published. So at this time there continues to exist a need for additional data of a favorable nature for our utilization and publication. Obviously to meet this need, studies will have to be accepted on a very selected basis, i.e., those known in advance to be favorable (pregnancy rate of 2% or less)."

Preston's search was in vain. She failed to find any favorable data suitable for publication.

Meanwhile, the medical profession's disenchantment with the Shield ballooned until it finally exploded in the congressional testimony of a young army doctor from Fort Polk, Louisiana.

Witness

*"Doctor, I thought I knew something about intrauterine devices,
but suddenly I have realized I knew less than I thought I did."*
—U.S. Representative Clarence Brown during
congressional hearings on the safety of IUDs, May 31, 1973.

Dr. Russel Thomsen missed the call when it came in to his office at the
Fort Polk Army Hospital in Louisiana in the middle of May 1972. Later,
his secretary told him the caller had been someone from Congress. She
didn't get a name or number.

"Gold something" was the best his secretary could do as Thomsen
pressed for the caller's name. He finally picked up a phone and, with luck
and the help of a knowledgeable Capitol Hill operator, was connected to
Gilbert Goldhammer, a consultant with the House Intergovernmental
Relations Subcommittee.

Goldhammer, who had long been involved in setting up the subcommittee's hearings on various medical issues, had come across several
letters Thomsen had written to the Food and Drug Administration
sharply critical of the Dalkon Shield. Hearings were set to begin in a week
on the need for federal legislation to strengthen control over medical
devices. The first hearing was to focus on IUDs, and Goldhammer
wanted Thomsen in Washington, ready to testify on the opening day.

"You really don't want me," an incredulous Thomsen said, "I'm just
out of residency. I'm nobody. I just wrote a couple of letters. Get the
experts."

To which Goldhammer replied, "Don't worry, when you testify, you'll be instantly an expert."

Thomsen, a major in the Army Medical Corps, spent a long and intense week in the small, limited medical library at the army base, pulling together research reports on IUDs and preparing his testimony. He already knew a great deal about the Dalkon Shield, for he had spent the last several months waging a one-man letter-writing campaign against the device. In addition to the FDA, he had written to the Federal Trade Commission and to A. H. Robins in an effort to find out everything he could about the Shield and the claims being made for it. Medical studies and other material he'd received from the government and A. H. Robins, information he had hoped would allay his fears, had produced just the opposite effect. He was now convinced the Shield was dangerous and should be pulled off the market.

It was a dramatic about-face for a military doctor who, during his residency two years earlier at the University of Utah Planned Parenthood clinic in Salt Lake City, had inserted hundreds of IUDs. Thomsen had gone to medical school in the late 1960s and had graduated without the bias against IUDs that was common among older physicians. The modern, plastic IUDs made sense to Thomsen, especially given the ongoing furor in the medical profession over the Pill.

It was while he was at the Planned Parenthood clinic that Thomsen first became familiar with the Dalkon Shield. A detailman from A. H. Robins approached Thomsen and began to talk about the new IUD. The detailman was personable, the son of a doctor, and equipped with very impressive statistics about the Shield. He pulled out graphs comparing it favorably to other IUDs on the market and quoted extensively from Hugh Davis' original study of the Shield. He did not, however, give Thomsen a copy of the full study. The device looked good in the drawings and its design seemed logical, Thomsen thought. It looked as though it had been made to fit into the uterus and it was supposed to be easy to insert. Why not try it?

Thomsen was one of many doctors in the family planning clinic at the University of Utah Medical School and at the nearby Latter-day Saints Hospital who had heard the pitch from the A. H. Robins detailmen. Soon almost all of the doctors were routinely inserting the Shield in their patients who wanted contraception. There were complaints of pain and bleeding from women during and after insertions of the Dalkon Shield and other IUDs, but Thomsen, like many of his colleagues, reacted indifferently. Indeed, Thomsen's initial reaction to the Shield was good. It seemed to be what the detailmen claimed it was—a superior IUD. His enthusiasm for IUDs, and the Shield in particular, allowed him to dismiss the complaints as insignificant.

In July 1972, Thomsen completed his residency at the University of Utah Planned Parenthood clinic and returned to active duty with the Army. Within a month, he was posted at the hospital at Fort Polk.

Almost immediately he was confronted by what he could only describe as a crisis—six women, all pregnant and all wearing Dalkon Shields. This is a very small hospital, he thought, and doctors at the facility couldn't have inserted the Shield in more than 150 women at most. To have six women who had become pregnant while wearing the Shield show up at the clinic at the same time was way out of proportion with anything Thomsen had ever seen. But the women were there, and they were all experiencing complications.

One of those women was Thomsen's nurse, who became pregnant four months after another doctor inserted her with a Dalkon Shield. She had a spontaneous miscarriage six weeks into the pregnancy. Another patient, the first of the Dalkon Shield women he saw, was upset because her previous physician, unable to find a cause for her repeated episodes of pelvic pain, had referred her to a psychiatrist. She had been told that her pain was "unreal" and would go away. Thomsen found a mass in the woman's pelvis, took her to the operating room, and discovered she had a ruptured ovarian pregnancy—a life-threatening condition.

Thomsen remembered the claims the A. H. Robins detailman had made for the Shield, so he looked again at the advertising material for the device. This time, however, he examined it with a critical eye and was appalled by what he saw. On October 9, 1972, only two months after arriving at Fort Polk, the once enthusiastic proponent of IUDs was so angered by what he was seeing in his patients and reading in the advertising material, that he wrote to FDA Commissioner Charles Edwards: "Having just worked through the past evening delivering another infant along with the omnipresent DALKON SHIELD," Thomsen began, "I am finally motivated to write the letter which I have considered for some time."

He told Edwards about the unusually high pregnancy rate associated with the Shield, as well as problems from excess bleeding. He listed eight serious side effects, including pelvic inflammatory disease, tubal pregnancies, and uterine perforation that he'd seen with the Shield and other IUDs. "Intolerable side effects occur in at least 30 percent of the users of IUDs," he wrote. As for the Dalkon Shield, Thomsen urged that it "be taken from the market until its safety can be proven (and not by company supported tests alone)."

It was the beginning of a determined, months-long effort by Thomsen to challenge the fashionable belief in the medical profession that IUDs were the near-perfect solution to contraception. And now, thanks to his effort, Thomsen had the ultimate forum—a congressional hearing, complete with national press—to make his views known.

No doubt his resolve to testify was strengthened when, as he was hurriedly preparing his testimony, another pregnant woman wearing a Dalkon Shield walked into the Fort Polk clinic. She became Thomsen's seventh such case in less than a year.

At 10:15 A.M. on May 30, 1973, Representative L. H. Fountain banged down his gavel in the spacious hearing room in the Rayburn House Office Building, and the Intergovernmental Relations Subcommittee hearing was under way.

"These hearings have been made necessary by reports in the medical literature and in the lay press of a mounting number of injuries and deaths resulting from devices which are found to be dangerous, defective, ineffective, or improperly installed," Fountain said as witnesses and reporters settled into their chairs. In the following months his subcommittee would look at the dangers of pacemakers, heart valves, impact resistant eyeglasses, and other medical devices, Fountain said. But the next few days were dedicated to revealing the problems caused by IUDs and the apparent inability—or unwillingness—of the federal government to regulate them.

Fountain, a friendly, drawling Democrat from Tarboro, North Carolina, was a 20-year veteran of Congress. He was truly upset over the reports of deaths and injuries caused by IUDs and wanted to know why they had happened. He couldn't understand how "those things" had gotten on the market without first receiving federal approval. But the problems the government had in regulating the devices would come later in the hearings. Today was the day to lay out the case against IUDs.

Goldhammer and his boss on the subcommittee staff, Delphis Goldberg, knew the critical tone of the testimony Thomsen and John Madry, Jr., an obstetrician and gynecologist from Melbourne, Florida, were about to give. Goldberg, a long-time veteran of congressional hearings on health issues, knew this hearing was going to be "a live one."

How live depended, of course, on the press coverage, and attracting much attention was going to be difficult. Senator Sam Ervin's special Watergate hearings had been under way for about two weeks and were dominating the news, and the Nixon Administration was embroiled in a heated dispute with Congress over the bombing of Cambodia. Indeed,

Representative Fountain was missing a special meeting on the War Powers Act so the IUD hearings could begin on time. Goldberg noted that at least there were a few reporters in the room—and one was from the influential *Washington Post*.

So the stage was set for the testimony to begin. First up was Madry, who had been conducting an anti-IUD campaign similar to Thomsen's. In his letter-writing campaign Madry, unlike Thomsen, had not directly attacked the Dalkon Shield or any other IUD by name. He was strongly opposed to all of the devices and criticized them as a group.

When the Pill, Madry's favorite method of contraception, came under siege in 1970, he had been pushed by demanding patients and the new anti-Pill momentum in the medical field toward IUDs. But Madry wanted to know more than the advertising brochures were telling him about the devices. He was especially interested in their mortality rates. So he began a personal survey, writing letters to 12 organizations, including Planned Parenthood; the World Health Organization; the Department of Health, Education, and Welfare; and several manufacturers of IUDs. None of them could tell him the death rate associated with the use of IUDs.

In the absence of hard data, Madry told the committee, he had called for the FDA to at least send a letter to all doctors warning them of the potential dangers of IUDs. He also asked for the federal government to conduct "reliable, unbiased studies" of IUDs. The studies might confirm, he said, "the increasingly convincing evidence that IUDs are unacceptedly hazardous for use by private physicians caring for private-pay patients." Trying not to be entirely negative in his assessment of IUDs, Madry said such unbiased studies "might provide the basis for a supportable argument that the IUD is at least safer than pregnancy itself and thus . . . beneficial to global efforts at population control."

By mid-morning Madry had completed his condemnation of IUDs and had set the tone for the hearings. His testimony served as the perfect introduction for Thomsen, who was about to launch a relentless attack on IUDs in general and the Dalkon Shield in particular. Thomsen would also offer some criticism, although relatively mild, of the FDA.

Goldberg knew the criticism was coming, and that by giving it, Thomsen was sticking his neck out. Thomsen's military superiors in Washington were not enthusiastic about an officer going before Congress on his own and criticizing a federal agency. Goldberg had had to make a few phone calls to the Pentagon to ensure that Thomsen would be allowed to testify.

To make sure everyone understood he was speaking as an individual physician, not a major in the Army Medical Corps, Thomsen included a disclaimer at the beginning of his written testimony: "The opinions or assertions contained herein are the private views of the witness and are not to be construed as official or as reflecting the views of the Department of the Army or the Department of Defense."

Thomsen, like Madry, was introduced to the subcommittee merely as a "concerned physician." He was a bit nervous as he sat down to testify and feared he might have to rush through his statement, for earlier that morning a subcommittee aide told him to be "very brief." The subcommittee was very busy, the aide had stressed, and he could only count on 15 to 20 minutes to testify.

Thomsen began his testimony by producing an assortment of IUDs for the five congressmen who sat before him. "I would just like to state," he said, "that I think in general that gentlemen have no idea what we are talking about when IUDs are mentioned, where they go, how much it hurts to have one put in, what a menstrual cramp feels like, and all of these other things." It might help, Thomsen said, if the congressmen could actually look at the devices they were talking about. "You can pass these back and forth and then keep them," he said as he handed them a nulliparous Dalkon Shield still attached to the end of an inserter, four sizes of Lippes Loops, a LEM (a four-legged IUD named after the space program's Lunar Excursion Module), and a Majzlin Spring.

Thomsen had organized his testimony into several sections, each detailing a particular complication caused by IUDs. He began with the high pregnancy rate of IUDs.

"IUDs allow unwanted pregnancies," he said, "which are more frequent and disastrous than the false advertising and misleading statistics of IUD promoters and manufacturers would indicate. But what is more important to the physician and his patients is the disastrous nature of IUD-incurred pregnancies." These "dire consequences," he continued, "are absolutely omitted from any mention in either advertising for the medical profession or patient information pamphlets put out . . . by the drug companies or by such organizations as Planned Parenthood."

Medical investigators had found that 40 to 60 percent of the pregnancies that occur with IUDs in place "terminate in spontaneous miscarriages," Thomsen said. "That certainly corresponds with my experience." And these IUD-caused miscarriages were more than "simple statistics on someone's textbook or paper. This is a miscarriage which the woman does not seek. The major portion of these miscarriages are serious medical emergencies requiring surgical completion with or without anesthesia, frequently the transfusion of whole blood, and often the use of massive doses of antibiotics because of infection within the incomplete miscarriage."

Thomsen next turned his attention to the pain caused by inserting an IUD, particularly the Dalkon Shield. "The A. H. Robins Company—in its information brochure for Dalkon Shield users—for the patients—condescendingly allows that 'some women have cramps for a short time after insertion, but these are generally mild and usually pass in a few minutes.' The general dismissal of pain in the brochure is definitely misleading and borders on falsehood," Thomsen said. "The person who wrote that was probably a man and most certainly had never undergone the experience of receiving a Dalkon Shield. I have seen a number of women faint following IUD insertion and particularly from Dalkon Shield insertion," he said.

Removal of the devices wasn't any better. Many women, remembering the pain of insertion, became so apprehensive at the prospect of removal that they asked "to be put to sleep during that fateful event," Thomsen said. "In fact, pain medication, a lead bullet to bite on, and a short memory are the requisites of some IUD removals, particularly the Dalkon Shield."

Thomsen next spoke of a "significant IUD complication" that is "studiously ignored in medical literature and is certainly omitted from any literature printed by IUD manufacturers for their women customers to read."

The complication was the "excessive number of X-rays which must be taken of women's abdomens or pelvis to localize misplaced or lost IUDs," he said. When an IUD tail string is not visible and a woman cannot verify that the device has been expelled, Thomsen said, an X-ray to locate the IUD is usually taken. The tail string can disappear for several reasons, he continued, pulling out X-rays to show the congressmen what he meant.

The Lippes Loop is prone to turning upside down in the uterus, he said, pulling the tail string up through the cervix. He told of instances where tail strings had been intentionally cut very short by physicians and were difficult to see. "It is an unfortunate commentary on the medical profession," he said, "but it is nonetheless true that some physicians purposefully cut the IUD string off so short that the patient cannot remove it [and so] it will be difficult for another physician to do so."

While it was difficult to come up with a figure on how many IUD-related X-rays were taken each year, Thomsen said, "I would think a good figure would be 10 per 1,000 IUD insertions." If there are two million women inserted with IUDs, he said, that would mean 20,000 women are "being exposed to pelvic X-rays a year in the United States for no other reason than to localize IUDs. I am sure that no one can calculate the genetic harm or carcinogenic harm done to American women and future generations by the yearly exposure of 40,000 ovaries to X-ray. But only a fool would claim that those X-rays are good for the ovaries and the eggs they produce."

Next on Thomsen's list were the problems of excessive bleeding and pain during menstrual cycles by women who wore IUDs. Excessive bleeding both during and in between periods was the most common reason for patients to ask to have their IUD removed, he said. About 20 percent of the women who received IUDs had them removed within two years because of bleeding, Thomsen said, and for every two that had them out, there is another woman who should because of a dangerously low blood count. "Within the last month," he said, "I saw a patient who insisted on retaining her Dalkon Shield even though she was required to take four iron tablets a day to maintain a minimally acceptable blood count."

In addition to heavy bleeding, Thomsen said, many women had excessive, persistent uterine cramping that his patients often compared to "having a baby each month." Many women take pain medication, even narcotics, in their effort to retain their IUDs, he said.

As for the claims by several pharmaceutical companies (including A. H. Robins) that IUDs allow women more freedom to enjoy sexual relations, Thomsen said, "Let me forever debunk this myth. For every woman who claims that her IUD has increased the enjoyment of her marital bed, I can quote two or more whose prolonged menses, unpredictable bleeding, and pelvic pain have either lowered the satisfaction of the sexual experience or basically compelled her to refrain from sexual expression."

Finally, Thomsen turned to the most serious consequences of wearing IUDs: critical illness and death. "Any clinician who has had adequate exposure to IUD patients and the complications they can have," he said, "will admit that he has seen one to several patients whose complications from the IUD would have led inexorably to death, if the heroic procedures and drugs of modern medicine had not intervened. Within the past year I have personally treated two such patients."

The life-threatening complications caused by IUDs, he said, were:

- Acute pelvic infection directly associated with IUD insertion.
- Acute pelvic infection with an IUD in place, but not related to the insertion.
- Perforation of an IUD through the uterine wall into the abdomen.

114

- Pregnancy with an incomplete miscarriage, usually requiring surgical completion, occasional blood transfusion, and possible use of antibiotics.
- Incomplete miscarriage with septic infection.

These complications certainly existed, Thomsen said, but there was no way a woman, reading the drug company promotional material or listening to her doctor quote from it, could determine what her chances were of developing one of these complications.

Another myth of IUDs, he said, is the claim that they are less expensive than other forms of contraception. IUDs, he said, have hidden costs. "The average IUD user bleeds over twice the amount each month than the normal woman or prior to the IUD insertion," he said. "This means that her monthly tampon or perineal pad bill is twice that of normal women."

The IUD woman might use iron pills to keep her blood count up, he said, and must also take occasional or regular pain medicine for IUD-induced cramps. The Dalkon Shield recommends some use of a spermicidal foam in addition to the IUD, and that costs money. Then there are the costs of treatment for infections, X-rays, a new IUD if the old one is expelled. The list of hidden costs continued through the significant expense of emergency surgery should one of the more serious complications develop. "It is interesting to me that most people or organizations which promote IUDs because of their inexpensive nature are universally unknowing or unconcerned about these common and major added expenses," he said.

Thomsen moved on to a section of his statement that, on his written copy, he'd entitled, "There is more than altruism in the sale of IUDs." Selling IUDs was a multimillion-dollar business for drug companies, he told the subcommittee. The devices cost 35 to 40 cents to manufacture, sterilize, and package, and were being sold to doctors for markups of about 1,000 percent, Thomsen said. "And that markup has come with little or no expenditure by the manufacturer for medical testing of the safety of its product. It might appear callous, but it's true, the name of the game in the IUD industry is profit."

A quorum call from the floor of the House interrupted the hearings about 20 minutes past noon, and Representative Fountain called a recess. Thomsen's initial nervousness had long since passed and by now he was enjoying himself.

Until this point, Thomsen had criticized the Dalkon Shield as part of a larger problem, but when the hearings resumed about 2 P.M., he turned his full attention to the device that had caused the "crisis" at his Fort Polk clinic. "Possibly no other IUD has received the benefit of such ecstatic claims by its developer, its manufacturer, and the admiring multitude," he said.

Thomsen told the congressmen that he had, "no personal vendetta against the Dalkon Shield or its manufacturer or promoter, who I have never met, or the company, one of whose medical directors has supplied me with considerable information. But I think . . . the Dalkon Shield and its promotion provide the classic example of the misuse of statistics to market an item." Both detailmen and printed advertisements for the Shield said one of the benefits of the Shield was that it was designed for the "average uterus." The eight-page progress report ad, for example, recounted how Hugh Davis and Robert Israel injected silicone into several "excised" uteri to determine their inner dimensions. They averaged the numbers and came up with, according to the ad, "the only IUD which is truly 'anatomically engineered' for optimum uterine placement." What no one seemed to recall, Thomsen said, is that "in human biology the average is merely an illusion. No one would think of producing the average brassiere and expect its use by basically all women. And few of my patients responded to their Dalkon Shield insertion as if their uterus knew it was average."

The more serious issue for Thomsen, however, was the validity of the four studies A. H. Robins was using to promote the Shield in its eight-page progress report advertisement. A. H. Robins, like other pharmaceutical companies, was promoting its IUD with "pathetic statistics," Thomsen charged. Calling it the "crux" of his testimony, Thomsen explained to the subcommittee how the statistics showing low pregnancy rates were derived from the "life table" method.

He explained how the life table method was invented specifically to gather statistics on IUDs. How it was designed to come up with statistically significant numbers on pregnancy and complication rates for these devices. And how it allowed investigators to draw statistics from a constantly changing group of women, for investigators apparently found it difficult to keep track of IUD wearers for long periods of time. This method allowed them to project statistically the long-term effect of IUDs on women without ever actually having to do a long-term study. At first glance life table statistics made IUDs look good, he said, but the way those statistics were gathered was "designed by those who are unabashedly promotional for IUDs, and therefore, it leaves out many complications that should have been included."

116

The life table method, he said, was a valid way to "draw some sense out of IUD research and statistics, but now it has been taken and incorporated into advertising. It was never even designed to be used for that." To show how a life table could mislead, Thomsen referred to its use by A. H. Robins in citing the four Shield studies in its progress report. "These studies were shown to cover from 9 to 12 months observation time," said Thomsen. "For example, Dr. Davis' study was 12 months, but the average insertion time was 5.5 months. In other words, the scratching for the forehead was done over 12 months, but the average insertion time was only 5.5 months." The life table method allowed A. H. Robins to say that the four studies totalled 17,222 women-months of Dalkon Shield usage. "For those who stop to make the calculation, however, it can be seen that the four studies actually involve the pathetic average insertion time of only 5.4 months," Thomsen pointed out. "In other words, the average patient in those four studies had her IUD Dalkon Shield for only 5.4 months. And buried in the small print footnote near the end of the ad was the recommendation that the patient should use another contraceptive along with the Dalkon Shield for up to the first three months post-insertion."

Thomsen also testified to his disagreement with the conclusion of a November 29, 1972, FDA memo written following a review of Dalkon Shield advertising after another IUD manufacturer complained about some of A. H. Robins' claims for the device. In the memo, David Link, director of the FDA's Office of Medical Devices, told Mervin Shumate, chief of the FDA's Bureau of Drugs, that there might be a few statements in the Dalkon Shield advertising that "fall into the mild puffery category. Otherwise, the information provided seems to be reasonable and accurate." In fact, Link wrote, the Dalkon Shield advertising seemed to be more complete than ads for other IUDs.

"I will agree that there are worse advertisements," Thomsen responded after Representative Fountain read the memo; but the memo missed a key point. "When this advertisement was written," Thomsen said, "A. H. Robins had far more studies available to it in its files that it disregarded and put in only favorable studies." Thomsen reached for his briefcase and, after sorting through its contents, pulled out a letter that had been sent to him by Ellen Preston, A. H. Robins' medical director in charge of monitoring the Dalkon Shield. Preston enclosed in the March 26, 1973, letter, a list of 11 studies, including the four used in the advertisement, that had been done on the Shield. The material, Thomsen said, showed that A. H. Robins, "in a calculated manner, definitely took four studies which I hold to be inadequate, the four very best studies, and put them in their advertisements while ignoring in their files studies which showed unacceptable complication rates."

Representative Fountain asked about the textbook on IUDs that had been written by Davis, a book that Thomsen had already described as a "thinly disguised promotion" of the Dalkon Shield.

Fountain turned to Appendix "A" in the book, which featured a chart that Davis had developed to show the comparative pregnancy, complication, removal, and expulsion rates for 10 IUDs. The Dalkon Shield, modestly listed last in the chart, was superior in every category.

Fountain took Thomsen through the chart, line by line. An IUD called the Small Gynecoil had a complication rate of 55.7 percent—"A disaster," Thomsen responded. Three other devices had complication rates ranging from about 41 percent to nearly 50 percent—"Totally unacceptable," Thomsen said. And so it continued, until Fountain reached the Dalkon Shield.

"Now, Dr. Thomsen," Fountain said, "The Dalkon Shield is shown . . . with only 5.4 percent total complications. From these data, would you regard the Dalkon Shield as safe and effective?"

"That is an amazingly effective device . . ." Thomsen answered. "That would have to be assumed to be a safe device."

How then, Fountain asked, could Thomsen reconcile the favorable numbers with his harsh criticism of the Shield? Remember that Davis was a co-developer of the Shield, Thomsen responded, and the 5.4 percent complication rate was based on an inadequate study of 640 patients who, on average, only wore the Shield for a few months. The figures for other IUDs in the chart, Thomsen said, were based on much larger and longer studies. Nowhere, he said, is that indicated on the chart.

"In other words, this is an amazing table," Thomsen said. "The deception is amazing."

At this point, Representative Clarence Brown jumped into the exchange between Fountain and Thomsen.

REPRESENTATIVE BROWN: "You think Dr. Davis then is party to fraud in the advertisement [in which A. H. Robins cited Davis' study]?"
THOMSEN: "Well—"
REPRESENTATIVE BROWN: "Well, you might as well say."
THOMSEN: "Yes, I do after going from the beginning to the end of this."

Thomsen's testimony had its most immediate impact 100 miles south of Washington at the A. H. Robins headquarters in Richmond, where company executives—including Jack Freund and William Zimmer—quickly gathered to discuss the army major's charges and how to respond. Although Thomsen had written to A. H. Robins detailing his problems with the Shield prior to testifying and had received a lengthy reply from Preston, A. H. Robins executives didn't know who he was or why he had so strongly attacked their IUD. Who was this guy, they asked themselves, and what did he want? What were his motives? Jack Freund thought Thomsen, as a young doctor, had been "spouting off" before the subcommittee without the expertise or data to support his statements. The company should appear before the subcommittee and respond to Thomsen, Freund told Zimmer and the other executives at the meeting. The officials agreed that their best response would be to appear before the subcommittee. And, as Freund had made the suggestion, he ought to be the one to go and testify.

When reporters phoned A. H. Robins in the early evening hours after Thomsen completed his testimony, the company responded strongly, rejecting Thomsen's charges out of hand and offering to go before Fountain's subcommittee and answer the allegations. It was not an offer made lightly, for no pharmaceutical company had voluntarily appeared before the subcommittee since it had begun its oversight of the FDA and medical issues in 1964. Fountain promptly took A. H. Robins up on its offer, and 13 days later, on June 12, 1973, Jack Freund, Ellen Preston, Donald Ostergard, Ken Moore, and H. Bradley Wells, a biostatistician from North Carolina, found themselves sitting in room 2154 of the Rayburn House Office Building. It was, Goldberg recalled later, a "high-powered crew" from A. H. Robins whose objective, he suspected, was to "try to perfume things."

Freund found the appearance "anxiety provoking." It reminded him of the nervousness he'd experienced years earlier when he'd taken his oral exams in medical school. Now, as then, Freund didn't know what to expect. But it wasn't what the congressmen asked that bothered him so much as it was the men behind them, the staff people who were constantly leaning forward and whispering questions to the congressmen. The staff members who did most of the whispering, and finally asked questions directly of Freund, were Goldberg and Goldhammer.

At about 10:30 A.M. the hearing started and Freund began his upbeat statement, telling the congressmen that the Dalkon Shield was an excellent product, with more than two million sold in the United States in its

119

first two years on the market. The Shield was the "IUD of choice" among a majority of ob-gyns who responded to an independent survey commissioned by A. H. Robins, he said. The Shield was being sold in 41 countries, he continued, and each component of the device was "quality assurance tested."

Freund only briefly turned his attention directly to Thomsen's charges of fraud in the A. H. Robins' advertisement promoting the Shield. "We view with grave concern the allegation made with respect to a particular Dalkon Shield ad," he said. "We categorically refute the charge of fraud and deceit in the selection of studies for citation in the ad."

In keeping with the A. H. Robins policy of citing only published studies in promotional material, the advertisement cited published studies he said.

Freund described the life table method of gathering statistics in terms that were remarkably similar to Thomsen's description of the method, saying it was "universally accepted by experts in the field and by professional journals and specifically endorsed by the World Health Organization." Freund did not, however, comment on Thomsen's complaint about the life table chart—that it was inappropriate for use in advertising a product.

A. H. Robins had changed the Shield for the better since acquiring it, Freund assured the committee. "The design was modified slightly for the purpose of facilitating insertion and removal and to minimize the incidence of pain and bleeding." The labeling was now clearer and more informative (including a detailed, four-page instruction sheet on how to insert the device without injuring the woman).

Freund failed to explain why A. H. Robins was using studies conducted with the original Shield to promote the newer, modified Shield. A. H. Robins had completed or was conducting extensive clinical studies, toxicity studies, and surveys of physicians, he said, all of which were generally favorable to the Shield.

After 1.8 million insertions of the Shield, he continued, A. H. Robins had received only 400 complaints, not a high number considering the number in use. Of course, Freund said, the company was responding to the complaints and considered them very important in considerations of future changes in the Shield. And raising a theme that would become one of the mainstays of A. H. Robins' defense of the Shield during the next 10 years, Freund said that some of the high pregnancy rates reported for the Shield were due, at least in part, to poor insertion techniques by doctors.

All in all, Freund offered a fairly brief, straightforward statistical defense of the Shield—a fine product put out by a fine firm.

Goldberg suspected A. H. Robins had come before the subcommittee thinking the appearance would give the company a platform for praising the Shield. Company officials may have expected the subcommittee to say thank you and goodbye after a few general questions, Goldberg thought; but he and Goldhammer, as well as Representative Fountain, had a different idea.

Fountain thanked Freund for his statement, then quickly challenged A. H. Robins' method of selecting medical data for use in advertising the Shield. Why, he asked, did A. H. Robins, seven months after Dr. Mary Gabrielson completed a study showing the Shield to have a 5.1 percent pregnancy rate, run an advertisement quoting only an earlier, abbreviated version of the study that showed the Shield with a 1.9 pregnancy rate? Why, Fountain asked, did A. H. Robins quote the 14.9 percent medical removal rate for the Shield from Gabrielson's early figures, but fail to mention the 26.4 percent removal rate in the final study? Why, Goldhammer asked, did A. H. Robins cite only these lower figures when it submitted its labeling to the FDA for approval a month and a half after Gabrielson had made her updated, more critical figures public?

Policy, Freund said, in A. H. Robins' defense. The company does not use unpublished studies in its advertisements, he said, and while Gabrielson had published the early results of her study, she had not published the final results. Freund admitted that Gabrielson had presented her final results in a paper at a national conference and that they had been published in *Family Planning Digest*. But that didn't count, he said, because the report had not been published in a scientific journal where it would be subject to peer review.

But what Freund didn't tell the subcommittee was that A. H. Robins had used unpublished data just a couple of months earlier in its March 1973 file card—not technically advertising—for the Dalkon Shield. "A composite of significant studies on the Dalkon Shield indicates a pregnancy rate of approximately 2%, an expulsion rate of around 3%, a medical removal rate of approximately 12%, and a continuation rate of about 80% at the end of 12 months," the card had stated. "These data are based on 11 studies in which some 20 investigators participated. The studies involve both multiparous and nulliparous women from clinic and private patient populations; include over 9,000 insertions; and represent 64,000 woman-months of use."

Most of those studies had not been published. Indeed, several had not even been "completed."

The heated exchanges went on throughout the morning as Freund,

Ostergard, and the other A. H. Robins representatives argued with Gold-hammer, Goldberg, and Fountain over what was and wasn't a valid study. The subcommittee adjourned just after 1 P.M., and Freund concluded that things had gone "very well."

That was not how Goldberg felt about it. "Gil Goldhammer and I felt we were getting a lot of bullshit," Goldberg recalled, especially from Ostergard and Wells, the biostatistician A. H. Robins had brought in from the University of North Carolina.

What was missing from Freund's testimony was any apparent concern for the women. He and the other company representatives easily recited the studies and statistics that supported the Shield and adroitly took apart studies critical of the device. But they didn't mention the seven pregnant women whom Thomsen had had to care for. They didn't say anything about the suffering of women with IUD-caused miscarriages, about the excessive number of X-rays many women with IUDs must undergo. They didn't talk about women fainting from pain following the insertion of the Dalkon Shield, or the emotional trauma of a young woman suddenly finding she was sterile because of the device. In fact, they hardly talked about the women at all.

But some women had listened, via the *Washington Post*, to the questions being raised about the Dalkon Shield. They knew firsthand of these problems, and they wrote to Fountain to tell him about them.

"I am twenty-seven years old, the mother of two sons, one 10 and one 9, and am the recent victim of the Dalkon Shield," wrote one woman. ". . . Before the first year with my IUD was up the pains were, at times, so intense that I was doubled over and could not straighten my body or walk correctly. This pain would encompass my body during the ovulation period and last for ten days to two weeks! Throughout all my visits to the doctor's office and my constant complaints, my doctor believed that it was due to the fact that I am a naturally hypertense person and that I was having [marital] problems, etc. It was felt that all this stress was causing my body to tighten up, hence the pain. I was given muscle relaxers."

Finally, no longer able to stand the pain, she went to the hospital and pleaded with her doctor to remove the device. An operation to remove the Shield failed, however, when the doctors couldn't find it. Four months later, an X-ray revealed that the Shield was exactly where it was supposed to be—in her uterus.

"I was never really told how this could be," the woman continued. "But my doctor gave some simple explanation which I really did not understand and we decided that since it was in the proper position, to leave it."

But the pain continued, and five months later another operation to remove the Shield was scheduled. "I was wheeled into the operating room for a *simple* D&C. I remember awakening and that there was a lot of confusion. Then I remember awakening again and discovered that I had been operated on. It seems that during the D&C the two doctors had tried to get the Dalkon Shield out and discovered that it had grown into the side of the cervical wall and that in the scraping process, while they were trying to dislodge the device, that an artery was severed and that this was not discovered until I had been brought up to the recovery room. When they discovered that I would hemorrhage to death, the only choice was to remove the uterus.

"I guess there is not much more to say. [It] is June 22, 1973 and I have yet to overcome the emotional impact of any of this, nor do I understand it . . . I guess the real problem is that I consented with my own free will—however, an uneducated, trust-in-my-doctor, free will."

According to former A. H. Robins attorney Roger Tuttle, there was considerable discussion among A. H. Robins executives about how to "neutralize" the impact of Thomsen's testimony following the hearings. But the company apparently did little to stop Thomsen from continuing to speak out against the Shield.

After the hearings, Thomsen received some hostile mail and phone calls from physicians, including some of his colleagues in the military. They accused him of needlessly worrying women and of not knowing how to properly insert Dalkon Shields. They believed he was part of another media event similar to the one that lead to the Pill scare.

Thomsen later learned that letters were written to two scientific journals trying to discredit him and to make it difficult for him to publish in those journals, but he declines to discuss the details of the letters or whom he suspects sent them. What these doctors didn't understand, Thomsen thought, was that the Dalkon Shield hadn't been thoroughly tested.

"IUDs, from that morning, were never the same," says Thomsen, now an army colonel, of his testimony after reviewing it 11 years later. "They weren't treated [the same] by the FDA, or by Congress, or by drug companies, or by physicians."

William Zimmer, who was shocked by what he felt was Thomsen's "belligerent" testimony about A. H. Robins and the Shield, also places significance on Thomsen's 1973 testimony.

"The beginning of our problems," he says, "were the Fountain Hearings and Thomsen."

12

The FDA

"Anyone—it doesn't even have to be a doctor—can go down to his basement, get a few hairpins, stick them together, and call it an IUD. There's nothing we can do about it until someone is injured or dies."

—Joseph Mamana, chief of the FDA's
Office of Medical Devices Compliance Section,
as quoted in the *National Observer*, September 8, 1973.

On May 25, 1973, only six days before FDA officials were scheduled to appear before Representative Fountain's subcommittee to explain how they were regulating IUDs, inspectors from the federal agency arrived at the doors of Anka Research Ltd., in Jamaica, New York. Once inside, they seized 9,000 Majzlin Spring IUDs, neatly packaged, 200 to a carton, for being unsafe. The Majzlin Spring, described by one doctor in a letter to Anka Research as an "instrument of the devil," was one of the inventions that had emerged from the IUD euphoria of the 1960s.

Because only about 100,000 Majzlin Springs had been sold, the device did not have the impact on women or on legislation that sales of the Dalkon Shield did. However, the Spring, which was first marketed in 1968, two years before the Dalkon Shield, did share many similarities with the Shield. It was a harbinger of things to come.

The Spring, like the Shield, was promoted to doctors as a modern and safe IUD, although doctors soon learned that it was anything but problem-free. The most common complaints against the Spring were that it perforated the uterus and that it was very difficult to remove.

The Spring, like the Shield, was sold to doctors and inserted in thousands of women without the device having gained the approval of the FDA or any other government agency.

And the Spring, like the Shield, was responsible for many horror stories from physicians and women, stories that the FDA gathered for several years before making any serious attempt to get the IUD off the market.

The Spring was developed and tested by gynecologist Gregory Majzlin at the State University of New York Downstate Medical Center's family planning clinic. It differed radically in design from previous IUDs. It was made of a long piece of stainless steel wire that folded and unfolded much like the bellows of an accordion. The device was compressed for insertion through the cervix, but once inside the uterus, it sprang open to its full shape. The folded wire configuration was designed to make the Spring very difficult for the uterus to expel. When the uterus contracted and pushed on the device, the Spring's top half would squeeze together, but the bottom of the device would expand, digging into the walls of the uterus. This kept the device from being pushed out, but it also caused serious cramps, bleeding, and uterine perforation. So many of the embedded or perforated Springs had to be removed surgically that Lillian Yin, the director of the FDA's Division of Ob-Gyn Devices, later said it seemed that "almost everyone who had it had a perforated uterus."

The seizure and subsequent recall of the Spring was the strongest action ever taken by the FDA against an IUD manufacturer. Unfortunately for many women, these actions came after the Spring had been on the market for five years. At the time of the seizure, the FDA announced in a press release that it wasn't certain how many of the Springs had been sold to physicians nor how many had been inserted into women. The best the FDA could say was that "over 100,000 of these contraceptive devices have been sold since 1968. The number in use is unknown." What the press release didn't explain was why the agency had waited so long to pull the Spring off the market.

The FDA was first alerted to the dangers of the Spring in 1970, three full years before the device was seized. Even stronger warnings of danger came in 1971, one of them in a letter from a doctor who told FDA officials that, given what was known about the dangers of the Spring, any physician using the device "is now essentially guilty of malpractice."

In both 1970 and 1971, the FDA responded to the complaints by inspecting the Anka Research facility. During the second inspection FDA officials found 39 letters in the company's files from physicians who had complained of serious problems with the device. The FDA didn't contact any of the doctors about the complaints and no action was taken as a result of the inspection.

Finally, in April 1973, after Representative Fountain sent his investigators to dig through the FDA's files to see how the agency was regulating IUDs, FDA officials decided to look a little harder at the Majzlin Spring problem. The Anka Research plant was inspected again, on April 10, 1973, the third time in as many years. This time FDA officials found new complaints from physicians and, in a report following the inspection, stated: "In reviewing this current report and the previous one, it is evident that many women are experiencing a great deal of discomfort, pain, torture, and serious injury due to use of the firm's IUD."

A month later, with the Fountain hearings only a few days away, the agency finally seized the Spring. Fountain called the timing "curious," and noted that all the FDA had really done was "put the finishing touches" on the demise of a product that was already being phased out of existence by its manufacturer because of mounting lawsuits and injury complaints. By the time the FDA moved, Fountain said, "the damage had already been done and many women . . . had been needlessly injured."

Russel Thomsen, in his testimony before the Fountain subcommittee, had addressed another critical issue raised by the Majzlin Spring case. The tens of thousands of women who had the Spring inserted, Thomsen said, "had no question but that the FDA had certified that these devices [were] not only safe but as wonderful as the promotional material asserts."

It was a reasonable assumption. After all, IUDs were being inserted by doctors at hospitals, clinics, and offices around the country. And the doctors, receiving most of their information from advertisements that praised the devices as superior, unique, modern and, in the case of the Spring, "new and improved," no doubt passed these glowing descriptions on to their patients—the women who had grown up in an era where all drugs, whether prescription or over-the-counter, required testing and FDA approval before being allowed on the market.

But the Spring, the Dalkon Shield, the Lippes Loop, the Birnberg Bow, and other IUDs on the market in the late 1960s and early 1970s were legally classified as "devices," not drugs—a crucial distinction of which few of the women injured by IUDs were aware. It was a distinction made in the Food, Drug, and Cosmetic Act of 1938, a law that was a breakthrough in its time and badly outdated by the end of the 1960s.

The FDA began regulating drugs in 1906, when the first general food and drug law banning interstate commerce of any adulterated or mis-

126

branded foods or drugs was passed. The 1906 law, known as the Food and Drug Act, did not regulate medical devices, however, and in the 1930s false therapeutic claims for quack devices were common in radio and newspaper advertisements. Reformers pushed for a law that would allow the FDA to go after those who sold quack devices in the same way the 1906 law had authorized the agency to pursue the makers of fraudulent drugs.

The result of the push to reform was the 1938 Act, which gave the FDA the power to regulate medical devices, for the first time—but only after they were on the market. The 1938 Act also strengthened the FDA's control over drugs, requiring that all new drugs be approved by the FDA "before" being sold. That approval provision did not apply to devices, however, because at the time most legitimate medical devices were fairly simple items such as orthopedic shoes, trusses, surgical instruments, and ultraviolet lights. Lawmakers apparently didn't see the need to have such devices cleared by a federal agency before reaching the public.

If a device proved to be dangerous once on the market, the "misbranding" provisions of the law empowered the FDA to remove it from the market—in common FDA parlance, to "seize" it. Under the provisions, any product, whether a drug or a device, could be ruled to be misbranded if it proved to be dangerous to public health even when used in the "dosage, or with the frequency or duration recommended or suggested in the labeling."

The FDA quickly used the law to pull from the market such dangerous items as lead nipple shields, which caused lead poisoning in nursing infants, stem pessaries, and an assortment of machines whose manufacturers claimed would cure a host of ailments with colored lights or electric current. But the 1938 Act left manufacturers free to design and sell any new medical device—without even having to inform the FDA of the device's existence.

As long as medical devices remained fairly simple, the 1938 Act seemed to take care of the occasional problem. But rapid technological advances in the late 1950s and early 1960s drastically changed the medical device field, and the 1938 Act quickly became antiquated. A law originally designed to protect the public from such things as lead nipple shields and trusses was, by 1970, the only law regulating such things as contact lenses, heart valves and pacemakers, kidney dialysis machines, and other highly complicated devices coming onto the market. Although many of these devices were critical to the health and safety of patients, under the 1938 Act none of them had to have FDA approval prior to marketing.

As long as a product was classified as a device, it was up to the government to prove that the product was not safe—after it was on the market. If a product was classified as a drug, however, the burden of proof shifted to the manufacturer to show that it was safe "before" marketing the product. In questionable cases, the decision on whether a new product was a device or a drug was left to the manufacturer. Although the FDA could challenge a product once it was on the market, the agency had a very difficult time keeping anything that could remotely be called a device from being sold.

The Majzlin Spring case, as FDA officials were quick to point out when questioned by Fountain in 1973, served to reveal the glaring inadequacies of the 1938 Act. The FDA had no power to check the Majzlin Spring before it was inserted into thousands of women, officials said. When the agency finally did seize the devices, it had to use the misbranding law, the same law used decades earlier to seize colored light machines that supposedly cured arthritis.

Thus, under the provisions of the 1938 Act, the Majzlin Spring was ruled to be misbranded in 1973 because it proved to be dangerous even when inserted and worn exactly according to the written instructions.

But while the Majzlin Spring incident showed the inadequacies of the law, it also showed that there was confusion, disagreement, poor communication, and hesitation inside the FDA in trying to regulate medical devices in general and IUDs in particular.

When Representative Fountain asked why the FDA, knowing of serious complaints against the Majzlin Spring as early as 1970, waited until mid-1973 to get the device off the market, FDA General Counsel Peter Hutt responded by outlining the FDA's regulatory approach to all IUDs:

"We never said these drugs or devices, whichever we will call them—these products—are without hazards. There are deaths, side effects, difficulties in insertion and in taking them out. The question is whether, again, particularly in view of the possible difficulties with other methods of contraception, whether the benefits outweigh the risks. Our conclusion has been up to this point that the benefits outweigh the risk, broadly speaking."

It was a conclusion that had been reached only after considerable disagreement within the FDA. It was also a decision reached as much for legal reasons as for medical ones.

In early 1968, at about the same time the Majzlin Spring was going on the market and Lerner and Davis were beginning work on the Dalkon Shield, the United States Court of Appeals for the Second Circuit ruled that a product used to suture severed blood vessels during surgery was a drug, not a device.

This was not the kind of ruling that attracts much attention from the public, but it was a very important decision for regulators in the FDA. Essentially, it gave the FDA a much stronger hand to regulate medical devices. It could also have changed the course of Dalkon Shield history—if FDA officials had used the power the decision gave them to take control of IUDs. And the agency almost did just that—but in the end, its fear of long and costly court battles with pharmaceutical companies won the day.

The court's decision, which went against AMP Inc., expanded the definition of a drug to include items that had been previously viewed as devices. The main consideration in determining whether something was a drug or a device, the court said, "must be the protection of the public health." The reason for the ruling, the court said, "was, very clearly, to keep inadequately tested medical and related products which might cause widespread danger to human life out of interstate commerce."

Soon after the decision, James Goddard, commissioner of the FDA, asked his general counsel, William Goodrich, how much power the ruling really gave the agency to regulate devices. Goodrich, who had been at the FDA for three decades, was one of the top authorities in the country on the 1938 Act.

In view of the court's liberal definition of what could be regulated as a drug, Goodrich told Goddard in a March 19, 1968, memo, the agency "should reconsider our regulatory policy concerning devices." Anything intended for long-term use in the human body, including IUDs, should be classified as a drug, he said. "Doubtful cases should be resolved in favor of classification as a drug." Goodrich's memo even included a three-paragraph statement detailing a new, tougher, regulatory policy and told Goddard it should be released.

One of the things that influenced Goodrich's recommendation to go after IUDs was a just-completed comprehensive report on the devices by an FDA advisory committee on obstetrics and gynecology. The report, published in January 1968, was generally favorable toward IUDs, but it did discuss "a definite, albeit small risk of infection and uterine perforation" caused by IUDs. The report included a survey of obstetricians and gynecologists in the United States, Canada, and Puerto Rico. Of the 6,443 who responded, 88 percent said they were unaware of any critical illnesses associated with IUDs—despite the report's estimate that two million women had been inserted with IUDs between 1962 and 1967 under generally unsterile conditions. The report did find 10 documented cases of death associated with the use of IUDs, but concluded that four of them were due to improper insertion procedures. "Serious adverse reactions associated with the IUD are rare," and often the result of faulty, unsterile insertions, the report concluded.

But Goodrich was concerned about the report's comments on adverse reactions, the problems with unsterile packaging and insertion techniques, and the need for more research and more adequate testing for IUDs. The AMP decision cleared the way for FDA to do something about IUDs, he said, and the agency should act. "I recomend [sic] the intrauterine device manufacturers be called to a meeting with you to discuss the steps to be taken for reasonably prompt filings of new drug applications," he wrote in the memo to Goddard.

In filing new drug applications, the IUD manufacturers would have to have their devices thoroughly tested to make certain they were safe. Devices already on the market would remain on the market but would be subjected to the same testing.

Goodrich was supported in his view that all IUDs should be reclassified as new drugs by both the director, Dr. Henry Simmons, and the deputy director, Dr. Marion Finkel, of the FDA's Bureau of Drugs, who were concerned about the "high incidents of adverse reactions" being reported about IUDs. But the meeting Goodrich wanted with manufacturers was never held, and IUDs stayed on the market.

While the court's interpretation of the AMP decision was helpful, it wasn't a substitute for what the FDA really wanted—a new law. The FDA wanted Congress to pass new legislation to update the 1938 Act and give the agency strong, pre-market regulatory rights over devices. Legislation strengthening device regulations had been introduced in Congress repeatedly throughout the 1960s, but had always died quietly. Some attorneys and administrators within the FDA thought Goodrich's proposal to summarily reclassify all IUDs as drugs would result in long, expensive court fights that would divert energy away from getting a new law through Congress. The more effective route, they argued, was to focus the agency's attention on obtaining new device legislation and to deal with IUDs on a case-by-case basis when problems arose.

On January 2, 1969, Goodrich wrote a memo to Dr. Philip Lee, assistant secretary for Health and Scientific Affairs at the Department of Health, Education, and Welfare, indicating that the idea of reclassifying IUDs as drugs still had momentum within the FDA. In the memo Goodrich said he had proposed that a new type of contact lens and a variety of IUDs be classified as "new drugs" on the basis of the AMP decision. The contact lens maker, Bausch and Lomb, had agreed to the new classification, he said, and "the IUD policy soon will be announced."

Starting with IUDs and new, soft contact lenses, Goodrich said, the FDA should use the AMP decision to gain regulatory control over the medical device industry product-by-product. But Goodrich acknowledged in his memo that, given the certainty of legal fights with many device manufacturers, development of the new policy promised to be expensive and time-consuming.

Nonetheless, the idea of using the AMP decision to regulate IUDs received a further boost within the agency in March 1969, when the medical advisory board to the FDA's Bureau of Medicine recommended tight regulation of IUDs. On April 9 Dr. B. H. Minchew, the acting director of the FDA's Bureau of Medicine, sent a position paper to W. B. Rankin, the deputy commissioner of the FDA, detailing the recommendations of the medical advisory board. The board had concluded that the FDA should take advantage of the AMP decision to "keep inadequately tested medical and related products with a potential for causing widespread danger to human life out of interstate commerce."

The best way to use the AMP decision to gain control of medical devices, the board said, was to single out IUDs as an example to the medical device manufacturers. The "FDA must seek to control the IUDs presently marketed and those under development," the position paper said. The cost of what amounted to reclassifying all IUDs as drugs was estimated by the Bureau of Medicine to be about $750,000 for extra staff, medical evaluations, and other implementation costs in 1970 alone.

As the FDA was struggling to figure out what to do with IUDs and other devices in 1969, another legal ruling reinforcing the AMP decision was issued, this time from the U.S. Supreme Court. The case involved the Bacto-Unidisk, a cardboard disk impregnated with eight different antibiotics. The disk was used to test for antibiotics that would be effective against various diseases. The Supreme Court ruled that the disk was a drug and said the definition of a device under the 1938 Act should be confined to such items as "electric belts, quack diagnostic scales and bathroom weight scales, shoulder braces, air-conditioning units, and crutches."

The AMP and Bacto-Unidisk cases gave the FDA unprecedented authority to reclassify devices as drugs without waiting for new legislation, but agency administrators and lawyers remained reluctant to use what they thought would be a long and costly legal approach to regulate devices. The ongoing device debate finally attracted the attention of HEW Secretary Robert Finch, who decided late in 1969 to establish a special "ad hoc" study group to determine what should be done. One of the major goals of the committee was to bring some order to the chaotic medical device field and pave the way for congressional passage of stronger laws. The study group was set up with Dr. Theodore Cooper, then-director of the National Heart and Lung Institute, as its chairman. Meetings were held with representatives of industry, doctors, consumers, and other government agencies. The committee conducted an extensive search of medical, industry, and government literature and found 10,000 injuries that were directly related to medical devices during the previous 10 years. Heart valves had caused 512 deaths and 300 injuries, the committee found. Pacemakers had caused 89 deaths and 186 injuries. Ten deaths and a startling 8,000 injuries were attributed to IUDs.

While the study wasn't exhaustive, Cooper said later, it did provide numbers from which conclusions could be drawn. In September 1970, the Cooper Committee released its report, which said that "problems do in fact exist and that a predictable increase in the complexity and sophistication of medical devices requires action now to prevent the emergence of even more serious and complex problems." The Cooper Committee recommended that devices be divided into three categories: devices such as bedpans and tongue depressors that need no standards or pre-clearance by the FDA; devices such as catheters and hard contact lenses that need meet only predetermined standards for design safety and manufacturing procedures; and devices such as cardiac pacemakers and heart valve replacements that must be cleared by the FDA prior to marketing. The committee also urged the FDA to begin sorting the thousands of medical devices on the market so they could be put into the appropriate categories. The FDA followed that recommendation; within a year a list of 8,000 individual devices being produced by 1,100 manufacturers had been compiled. By the end of 1972, the FDA had set up the Office of Medical Devices to deal specifically with the thousands of medical devices. It also established two panels of experts to begin classifying each of the thousands of devices based on its safety and efficacy.

It sounded good. The Cooper Committee recommendations had finally moved the FDA to action at a time when it was badly needed. But the recommendations of the Cooper Committee also had another effect. They overshadowed the earlier recommendations of Goodrich and the others within the FDA that all IUDs be classified as drugs. Exactly when the Goodrich recommendations were rejected is not clear, but Peter Hutt, the FDA's attorney at the time, takes responsibility for turning the agency away from the path suggested by Goodrich. "I was very clearly of the opinion that, because there was no legislation (classifying an IUD as a drug), it clearly was a device," Hutt said recently.

After the AMP and the Bacto-Unidisk decisions, Hutt said, FDA officials "asked me could we get away with declaring it [IUDs] a drug and I said clearly not." Hutt did not agree with Goodrich's interpretation of the court decision, and he felt that focusing agency efforts on trying to use the courts to regulate IUDs "would divert attention away from the issue, which was the safety [of the devices]." He urged the agency to put its efforts into classifying devices and getting new legislation through Congress. "My view was let's not get tangled up in the underbrush," said Hutt, who now advises pharmaceutical companies on the potential effect of federal government regulations. (Hutt said he has never represented A. H. Robins.)

While the FDA abandoned the idea of classifying all IUDs as drugs, it did make an exception for a new category of IUDs—those containing copper or other "active ingredients."

In 1968, Dr. Jaime Zipper, a physician from Chile, had demonstrated in tests with rabbits that adding copper to an IUD increased its contraceptive effectiveness. It was not clear precisely how the copper made IUDs more effective, but it was theorized that when the metal leached out of the IUD, it killed sperm. The FDA decided that the added contraceptive effect should qualify any IUD containing copper or other "heavy metals" as a new drug, subject to pre-market testing and approval. And in June 1971, the agency issued a proposal in the Federal Register saying that IUDs using "any active substance to increase the contraceptive effect, to decrease adverse reactions, or to provide increased medical acceptability, are not generally recognized as safe and effective for contraception."

Three types of IUDs were exempted from the proposal: those made from materials that did not interact with the body; those with substances added solely to improve physical characteristics (such as flexibility); and those containing a substance, such as barium, for the exclusive purpose of enabling the IUD to be seen by X-rays.

But it would be more than 20 months later, in late February 1973, before the FDA would make the regulation official. From that date on, IUDs with active ingredients were classified as drugs; those without were devices. Ironically, it was Dr. Marion Finkel of the FDA's Bureau of Drugs—the same Dr. Finkel who had worried that IUDs were dangerous and endorsed Goodrich's memo—who developed the agency's final position on IUDs.

For A. H. Robins officials, the FDA's announcement in June 1971 of its position on copper in IUDs could not have come as good news, but neither did it come as a surprise. More than a year earlier Finkel said that

A. H. Robins would be required to submit a new drug application for the Shield because of the copper it contained.

Finkel's recommendation that the Shield be classified as a drug was apparently ruled out in the ongoing regulatory debate within the FDA, but A. H. Robins officials certainly were concerned about the interest the FDA was showing in the copper content of their IUD. Company officials were aware that Lerner and Davis had added enough copper to the Shield that it turned blue-green with oxidation. The company was also aware of Davis' statement in *Good Housekeeping* that "with the addition of copper, the shield device is virtually 100 percent effective in preventing pregnancy." However, since Lerner and Davis hadn't bothered to conduct studies on the Shield after adding the copper, there was no way for A. H. Robins to really know if the copper enhanced its efficacy.

But there was Roy Smith's troubling memo, written in June 1970, about the "drug effect" of the copper and about how it might be misleading "not" to tell doctors that the copper had been added to the Shield "for the express purpose of getting a 'drug effect.' "

Early in the Shield's marketing campaign, some of A. H. Robins' detailmen had spoken to physicians about the contraceptive effect of the copper in the Shield. None of the Shield's promotional materials made mention of copper, however. And just before the FDA publicly proposed classifying IUDs with copper as drugs, the company ended all discussion of copper as a contraceptive in the Shield, instructing its detailmen—and Davis—to refrain from referring to the Shield's copper as a contraceptive agent. In April 1971, two months before the FDA issued its new IUD regulatory proposal, A. H. Robins' general sales manager John Burke sent a memo to company sales representatives that said, "In view of recent developments regarding the regulatory status of copper-containing intra-uterine devices, it is essential that you avoid any suggestion or implication that the copper additives contribute to, or enhance the contraceptive effectiveness of the Shield."

The company told the FDA that the copper was in the Shield only to give it more flexibility and strength and to make the device visible to X-rays; A. H. Robins argued that it should be classified as a device, not a drug, and exempted from any testing.

That A. H. Robins could convince the FDA that the Shield was a device was far from a sure thing. In October 1971, Ken Moore, A. H. Robins' project manager for the Shield, said in an in-house memo that the company didn't have much basis for telling the FDA the copper was added to improve the physical properties of the Shield. The copper "does not and never was intended to contribute to the above-mentioned properties [flexibility and strength]," he said. "Therefore we are in a very vulnerable position, in my opinion."

At about the same time that Moore was writing his memo, the FDA was sending out a letter to Charles Swartz, an attorney from Warren, Ohio, saying the Dalkon Shield had indeed been classified as a drug: "Dalkon Shield is regarded as a new drug . . . as set forth in the proposed statement of policy published in the Federal Register for June 5, 1971," wrote Peter Angeramo, an official in the Office of Compliance in the FDA's Bureau of Drugs. "We are unable to say when the final order of this policy statement will be published. Information submitted by manufacturers of new drugs . . . is regarded as confidential and may not be revealed."

Seven months later the FDA sent A. H. Robins a letter saying the Dalkon Shield was a device, not a drug. The FDA's final order on the classification of all IUDs did not go into effect until February 1973.

When asked by the Fountain Committee about the discrepancy between the October letter describing the Shield as a drug and its final classification as a device, Hutt said it was apparently the result of "a massive lack of communication within the agency." Hutt also said an FDA memo written on August 5, 1971, concluded, after a review of Shield data that had been supplied by A. H. Robins, that the possibility of the copper in the Shield increasing the device's effectiveness was "to be considered practically nil." The memo went on to state, Hutt said, "that there was no clinically significant difference between whether the copper was in there or not, and thus, apparently on the basis of this, the conclusion was made this was not to be classified as a copper IUD."

On May 4, 1972, the FDA made it official and sent a letter to A. H. Robins stating that, based on a review of data supplied by A. H. Robins, "we have concluded that Dalkon Shield, as labeled is a device."

Of course the material sent to the FDA didn't mention Roy Smith's concerns about the "drug effect" of the copper in the Shield. It would not be until 12 years later, in a courtroom in Minneapolis, that Smith's memo would finally be made public.

Getting the Shield classified as a device was clearly a victory for A. H. Robins. The company could continue marketing the Shield without testing and without the government looking over its shoulder.

But there was another, more serious problem about to descend on the company. Women wearing the Shield were experiencing severe and life-threatening infections—the kind of problems that might have been discovered in the clinical testing the FDA required pharmaceutical companies to conduct for new drugs, but not for devices.

13

The Shield Breaks

"I looked at the tail, and thereby hangs the tale."
—Howard Tatum, M.D., March 1985.

On March 30, 1973, a 31-year-old Arizona woman, the mother of two small children, died after her infected uterus spontaneously aborted the baby she had been carrying for more than four months. The infection had spread rapidly through her body, essentially poisoning her. Antibiotics and other desperate medical measures had not been able to save her.

This kind of septic abortion—one that occurs spontaneously in the middle trimester of pregnancy—was extremely rare in 1973. Up until that time, the only septic abortions doctors had seen were in women who had become infected during an illegal or self-induced abortion.

The young Arizona woman had not tried to abort her baby. She had, however, become pregnant while wearing a Dalkon Shield and was still wearing it when her pelvis became poisoned.

A. H. Robins officials learned of the woman's death two months later through the medical grapevine. A group of doctors at a Miami medical conference had been discussing how to treat sepsis when an Arizona doctor, Duncan Reid, mentioned the septic abortion death of the woman, who had been his patient. Word quickly spread in the medical community of the association between the septic abortion death and the Dalkon Shield. Soon doctors were talking of "several" or "seven" deaths among Shield wearers.

A. H. Robins wanted to know what was going on. So did the FDA, which had also heard the talk about women dying from the Shield. A. H. Robins officials tracked Reid down to the University of Arizona College of Medicine in Tucson, Arizona, and asked for more details about the woman's death, but Reid was apparently uncooperative. As Ellen Preston noted in a memo to her file: "[He] indicated that he did not intend to become further involved in this situation with us or the Food and Drug Administration. [He] said he found it very distasteful that the Food and Drug Administration would concentrate or attempt to single out any one IUD for particular action, because they all had their problems. . . . He furthermore felt that decisions as to patient management were matters for the practicing profession and not the FDA."

Reid considered the death of his patient, according to Preston, "only one isolated case and [it] could have but very little meaning of itself with respect to IUD use."

But it wasn't an isolated case, and it had a great deal of meaning for other women wearing the Shield. During the next few months of 1973, A. H. Robins would receive five more reports of women dying from septic abortions while wearing the Dalkon Shield. And the death toll continued to climb from there.

Reid was not the only doctor who delayed making such reports. Three of those first six reported cases involved women who had died in 1972. Why it took so long for all of these doctors to pass on this information to A. H. Robins or to the FDA remains an unanswered question. Although physicians are not legally required to contact the FDA about such matters, it is not unusual for doctors to do so.

"The majority of early reports came to us in round-about-ways," Fred Clark told the FDA in 1974, "with only a very few reported directly from a physician shortly following an occurrence."

A. H. Robins had, however, gotten a very direct report from Dr. Lindsay Curtis, a gynecologist from Ogden, Utah. Curtis had visited A. H. Robins' Richmond headquarters in June 1972 and told the company's officials that he and a group of physicians he worked with would no longer be using the Dalkon Shield. He had personally seen three cases of serious pelvic infections in Shield wearers—including one in a 25-year-old woman who had developed a severe infection and a temperature of 105 degrees before giving birth to a stillborn baby. That young woman was his daughter, Curtis added.

Ellen Preston wrote to Curtis a few days later: "Needless to say we were disappointed to hear that your experience had not been altogether favorable, particularly with regard to serious pelvic infection associated with Shield use. As I believe we indicated during our conversation, we have received other reports of PID occurring in Dalkon Shield wearers, but the reports have been very infrequent. I am sure, however, as you pointed out we do not receive reports on all the cases that occur."

Only a few days earlier A. H. Robins had received the letter from Thad Earl warning of the possible connection between the Shield and septic abortions and recommending that doctors remove the Shield from any patient who became pregnant while wearing it. But A. H. Robins failed to pass that recommendation on to doctors in its labeling for the Shield for almost 18 more months.

Nor was Earl the only A. H. Robins consultant warning the company about septic abortions. John Board at the Medical College of Virginia (MCV), had served occasionally as a consultant for the Dalkon Shield; and his wife, Dr. Anne Board, worked in A. H. Robins' medical services department. She had alerted the company early in the spring of 1973 to the concerns of her husband's MCV colleagues regarding the Shield.

"Dr. Leo Dunn and others at MCV have inquired (via John to me to you) about the problem of septic abortion associated with the Dalkon Shield," Anne Board reported in a April 16, 1973, memo to Ellen Preston. "As well as I can determine, there is a feeling or rumor (based upon the fact that several individuals have each experienced one case) that if a patient becomes pregnant while having a Dalkon Shield in place, therapeutic abortion should be carried out post-haste. The reason for this is that patients with Dalkon Shields are more likely to experience septic abortion than either (1) patients using other IUDs or (2) patients without IUDs who happen to experience spontaneous abortions."

A. H. Robins continued to treat these cases as isolated incidents, however, and didn't pursue them with much vigor for many more months. "I would estimate that I have been advised of a dozen, at the very most, cases of septic abortion associated with the Dalkon Shield," Preston wrote to John Board. "It is not necessary to point out—to you anyway—that all such events do not come to our attention, but at any rate we have not been besieged with reports of septic abortion."

The company was getting some angry, and anguished, letters from women who were personally experiencing the emotional and physical trauma of a septic abortion. One woman wrote that she had been "unlucky enough" to have a Dalkon Shield inserted in February 1972.

"Nine months later in December of the same year, I found myself pregnant," the woman reported. "I was advised by my doctor, at that time, that he could not remove the device (which had come out of place and was embedded in the wall of the uterus) without causing a spontaneous miscarriage. I was only 6 weeks along at this time, and could of, of course, had an abortion, but the fact was that when I found myself pregnant I wanted the child very much."

But the pregnancy lasted only five months.

"Without warning, on Easter Sunday, April 22, 1973, I became suddenly ill," the woman continued. "I was vomiting, had diarrhea and was running 104 temperature. I also had very mild contractions at this time. I immediately contacted my Doctor and was rushed to the Emergency Room. The Doctor suspected a kidney or bladder infection but blood and urine tests proved negative. I stayed at the hospital overnight, and the contractions became stronger, the Doctor gave me a drug to try and stop the contractions, but by 5:00 p.m. on Monday, it was clear that delivery was imminent. At 7:30 that evening my baby was born and immediately died. My doctor then removed your wonderful device, which had caused all the trouble. A study of the placenta showed that there had been an infection caused by [the Shield] and that was why blood and urine tests did not show any kidney or bladder infection."

After the delivery, the woman's temperature rose to 107 degrees, she reported, and she went into shock. "Thank God after five days in the hospital I did recover, that is physically," the woman concluded. "To this day I wake up with nightmares of that night."

By the end of 1973, the dam had broken and reports of deaths and severe cases of sepsis associated with the Shield were becoming more widely reported. A. H. Robins officials insisted, however, that the Shield was getting a bad rap, that it was no worse in this regard than any other IUD. Indeed, the Lippes Loop and Saf-T-Coil were soon associated with septic deaths, although not nearly as many.

Compounding the problem were new studies that revealed to doctors across the country what A. H. Robins already knew—that the Shield's pregnancy rate was much higher than the claimed 1.1 percent. In January 1974, a one-year study conducted at the Kaiser-Permanente Medical Center in Sacramento, California, was published in the *American Journal of Obstetrics & Gynecology*. It reported a 5.6 percent pregnancy rate among 296 Dalkon Shield wearers (and a high 28.7 percent removal rate for pain, bleeding, or other medical reasons).

"In our opinion," stated the study's authors, "the pregnancy rate . . . contra-indicates the use of the Dalkon Shield in nulliparous women unless local contraception is also used, particularly during the initial three months when failures tend to occur." Yet another study had been completed at the Beth Israel Hospital in Boston and was scheduled to be published in March 1974. It would report an astounding 10.1 percent pregnancy rate for the Shield.

Doctors were concerned. Not only was the Shield being linked to an unusual number of septic abortions, but it also was apparent that Shield wearers ran a greater risk of becoming pregnant in the first place.

The company decided something had to be done to clear the Shield's bad name—the decision took on even greater urgency when company officials learned in late 1973 that Donald Christian, a doctor in Tucson, Arizona, would soon be publishing a paper on the Shield and its relationship to septic abortions. Christian was head of the ob-gyn department at the University of Arizona Medical Center in Tucson—the same hospital where the 31-year-old woman had died after a septic abortion. Her death had puzzled him, as had two other deaths of Shield-wearing women he learned about from a Texas doctor several months later. One of these involved a 24-year-old mother of two who had become pregnant three-and-a-half months after being fitted with the Shield in January 1972. She developed flu-like symptoms during her fourth month of pregnancy—fever, nausea, sore throat, and vomiting. Three days later, after entering a hospital, she had a miscarriage. The following day, she died.

Christian says that after learning of these two additional deaths, he contacted the FDA and the Centers for Disease Control, but was ignored. He says he also contacted A. H. Robins. It is at this point that the story gets confusing, however. A. H. Robins officials insist it was *they* who contacted Christian after receiving reports in November 1973 that he had told a group of doctors in Acapulco of Dalkon Shield-related septic abortion deaths.

In any event, Christian and Ellen Preston had a tense telephone conversation on November 21, 1973.

"During the course of [our] 10 to 15 minute conversation," Preston wrote in a later memo, "Dr. Christian made the following points:

1. This information on deaths associated with the Dalkon Shield had been supplied to the President of our company way back in the spring of 1973.

2. The company had done nothing about the information and had assumed a very 'unstatesman like' attitude toward this very serious problem of sepsis and septic abortion with deaths associated with the Dalkon Shield.

3. Our salesman continued to pooh pooh and dismiss any information indicating there was any problem with the Dalkon Shield."

Preston then noted how she had replied to Christian:

"1. So far as I knew information supplied to us in the Spring came from Dr. Duncan Reid of his department and involved only one death associated with the Dalkon Shield.

NOTE: In reviewing Dr. Owen's notes on a phone call he had to Dr. Reid I see that Dr. Donald Christian's name is mentioned as head of the department. However, the note does not convey to me the idea that we should have gotten in touch with Dr. Donald Christian perhaps instead of Dr. Duncan Reid. Perhaps this is why Dr. Christian was so hostile."

2. I indicated to Dr. Christian that this information about the death Dr. Reid reported had been passed on to the FDA. Furthermore, revised labeling pointed out the problem of septic abortion and recommended consideration be given removing the Shield if pregnancy was diagnosed, etc.

3. For our salesman we attempted to keep problems associated with our products and in proper prospective [sic] as best we could on the basis of available information."

Preston also offered to follow-up on any reported cases of death. "I inquired as to whether the three deaths he had collected were all associated with pregnancy," she wrote. "He replied that was the whole point. I suppose that was intended to mean that I had asked a dumb question."

Preston did follow-up on Christian's report by visiting him in Tucson on December 10, 1973. She told Christian "that we wanted to do what was right about it and we needed his help." Christian told her that he had evidence of a link between the Shield and fatal spontaneous septic abortions.

She wrote up that meeting in a memo. "He brought up what he might do with the information he had," Preston wrote. "He intends to publish it, I think. . . . He pointed out that he could call the editors of several journals and get it published in their next issue with a black border around it, etc., and that would be the end of the Dalkon Shield."

A few weeks later, about the same time Christian submitted a draft of an article describing cases of septic abortions to a medical journal, A. H. Robins asked the FDA if it could present its own septic abortion data to one of the agency's advisory panels. But when the FDA put the company off, A. H. Robins officials say, the company decided to convene its own special conference on septic abortions.

A. H. Robins invited several well-known contraception specialists to serve on the conference's panels, including Howard Tatum, who was the inventor of the Copper-T IUD and at that time the associate director of the biomedical division of the Population Council; and Michael Burnhill, who was then the medical director of the Preterm Medical Clinic in Washington, D.C., and the inventor of the Birnberg Bow IUD. Donald Christian also came.

A. H. Robins also saw to it that the panels were well supplied with their own consultants. Hugh Davis was in attendance, although he was never identified as a consultant to A. H. Robins or as the recipient of royalties from the Dalkon Shield. Also participating in the conference were five members of A. H. Robins' Advisory Panel for Family Planning and Birth Control. These were the "troubleshooters" who had been hired during the Shield's second promotional blitz to spread the good word about the device throughout the country.

Noticeably absent from the guest list of this private, invitation-only event was Thad Earl, the doctor who had warned A. H. Robins about septic abortions in the first place. A. H. Robins had not invited Earl. Howard Tatum said later that he thought Win Lerner should also have been at the conference, as he was the person most familiar with the actual design of the Shield; but Lerner was absent, too.

The conference opened at 9:00 A.M. on February 15, 1974, in the auditorium of A. H. Robins' research building on Sherwood Avenue in Richmond. The room was equipped for taping, but A. H. Robins officials insisted that there be no taping during the conference. (Ten years later, in February 1984, Patricia Lashley, who worked as a secretary and then as a paralegal for A. H. Robins, testified in a deposition that a tape of the septic abortion conference existed. Two months later, she changed her mind and said the tape didn't exist.) Someone, however, must have taken copious notes, for a detailed summary of the panel discussions was later written and typed, with CONFIDENTIAL stamped on its front page.

Ellen Preston opened the conference by telling the doctors that A. H. Robins knew of 32 cases of sepsis or septicemia associated with spontaneous abortion in Dalkon Shield wearers; including five cases that had resulted in the deaths of the women. Preston stressed that this number should be kept in perspective with the more than 2.2 million Shields that had been inserted in women in the United States.

Preston then announced that A. H. Robins had recently changed its official labeling for the Shield to warn doctors that deaths from severe sepsis had been reported in women who had become pregnant and then spontaneously aborted while wearing the Dalkon Shield. (In this labeling, which was printed in October 1973, A. H. Robins told doctors for the first time that "serious consideration should be given to removing the device when the diagnosis of pregnancy is made with a Dalkon Shield in situ.") But there is some confusion about whether this new labeling was ever sent to doctors. A. H. Robins says it was; attorneys for women who later filed suit against the company say there are indications that the labeling never left A. H. Robins headquarters.

Preston and other company officials obviously wanted to convey the message that their company was doing everything possible to limit the risk of septic abortion in Shield wearers. They also wanted to make sure the Shield was not singled out as being more dangerous than other IUDs.

Frequently during the conference, a panelist would criticize the Shield specifically, only to be rebutted by a member of A. H. Robins' advisory panel. During one discussion, a doctor described the high rate of septic pregnancies he had observed in his Dalkon Shield patients and speculated that the device's design might have played a role in the sepsis. An A. H. Robins consultant quickly came to the Shield's defense, suggesting that perhaps these septic abortions were the result of infections that began outside the uterus. When yet another doctor told the group that his clinic had stopped using the Dalkon Shield because of concern about septic abortions, an A. H. Robins consultant told the story of a patient of his who had died after a septic abortion, but who had never worn any IUD at all.

The conference had other interesting—not to say ironic—moments. One doctor reminded the group that infections similar to those being discussed at the conference had occurred years ago with stem pessaries and suggested that perhaps "any foreign body" placed in the uterus could lead to infection. This warning, an old and an increasingly unfashionable one, apparently went unheeded, as it had so many other times over the years.

Hugh Davis participated in a panel discussion late in the day. When the Shield was criticized he came strongly to its defense, stating that none of his Shield-wearing patients had died from sepsis, nor did he know of any such cases in Baltimore.

Davis did acknowledge one case of sepsis in a patient of his who had become pregnant while wearing the Shield. But, Davis said, he learned later that she had tried to induce an abortion by inserting a catheter into her own uterus. That had obviously caused the infection, he said. Davis hinted that he felt many of the septic abortions being reported in IUD wearers were the result of women trying to abort their babies themselves. "Anyone who has studied abortion data recognizes the difficulty in obtaining the true facts from patients," he indicated, according to A. H. Robins' minutes of the conference.

(Of course, even if Davis' insinuations were true, he ignored the fact that the women would not have had to resort to this desperate act had they been told the Dalkon Shield's true pregnancy rate in the first place. They had, after all, chosen what their doctors said was a "superior" form of birth control—a claim based on the original study by none other than Hugh Davis.)

Surprisingly, it was Davis who first brought up the question of the tail string at the conference. Appendages from IUDs could very well be a "causative factor" in infection because body fluids could penetrate the tail string and create the environment for infection, Davis said. But this happened only with woven threads, he stressed. Neither Davis nor any of the A. H. Robins officials present in the auditorium bothered to tell the other doctors at the conference that the tail string of the Dalkon Shield was not a standard monofilament string, but a multifilament string that A. H. Robins was "desperately" trying to replace.

Howard Tatum left the one-day conference with more questions than answers. He felt he hadn't learned much at the meeting. Not enough information had been presented to really settle anything. At one point, some of the conference participants had actually voted on whether they believed that Dalkon Shield wearers were at a greater risk of sepsis than other IUD users. The vote had been indecisive: five "yes," five "no," and two abstentions.

Tatum was worried that all IUDs were getting blamed for something that might be unique only to the Dalkon Shield. He wanted to clarify the issue of the relationship between sepsis and IUDs before the use of these devices in family planning clinics throughout the world was threatened. Tatum was a strong believer in IUDs, especially in his own device, the Copper-T. (But unlike Davis, Tatum had no intention of making a profit from his invention. He sold all his rights to the Copper-T to the Population Council for one dollar.)

Tatum decided to take a closer look at the Dalkon Shield to see if it had any particular properties that made it more likely to lead to sepsis than other IUDs. It was during this examination that he discovered for the first time that the Shield's tail string consisted of several hundred separate fibers rather than a single or double strand of solid plastic thread, as could be found in the tail strings of four other IUDs—the Lippes Loop, Saf-T-Coil, Copper 7, and his own Copper-T. Maybe here lay the answer, he thought. Maybe the physical structure of the Shield's tail string functioned as a wick, drawing bacteria into the uterus.

Tatum began a wicking experiment. He suspended the tail strings of several Shields and of four other IUDs in a dye solution. Within 24 hours (and sometimes as quickly as two hours) the dye rose through the entire length of the Shield's tail string, passing through both knots. It did not ascend through the monofilament tails of the other devices. Tatum had found out what Lerner and Crowder had discovered before him—the Shield's tail string wicked.

But Tatum didn't stop there. He conducted another wicking experiment, this time immersing the tail strings in a saline solution containing live Escherichia coli bacteria, which are often found in the vagina. After 48 hours, he found that the bacteria had risen through the Dalkon Shield tail string all the way to the base of the final knot. When a woman wore the device, this knot would be well inside her uterus. No bacteria had ascended the other tail strings.

To confirm his findings, Tatum collected tail strings from Dalkon Shields, Copper 7s, and Copper-Ts that had been removed from women in clinics throughout the United States. He attempted to culture bacteria from the interior of these tail strings. He was successful, but only with the Shield. It was now his strong opinion that live bacteria from the vagina could and frequently did enter the spaces between the fibers within the sheath of the Dalkon Shield tail string.

But the bacteria had not been able to wick through the top knot of the string, and the tail string, after all, was surrounded by a protective sheath. How, then, did bacteria enter the uterus? Tatum offered his theory:

"An interesting observation was that many of the tails of Dalkon shields that had been sent to us for examination after their removal from patients had one or several breaks in the nylon sheath. Although these holes were encountered at various locations throughout the length of the tail, they commonly were seen in the sheath immediately below the double knot at the base of the shield. It is not illogical to postulate that microorganisms that had gained access to the interfilamental spaces through the open end of the tail in the vagina could migrate upward and exit through a break in the sheath into the endometrial cavity."

This, of course, is exactly what Wayne Crowder had speculated three years earlier when he had first noticed breaks in the sheath. Howard Tatum began to write up his findings for publication.

In June 1974, Donald Christian's devastating article on the connection between the Dalkon Shield and fatal cases of sepsis appeared in the American Journal of Obstetrics & Gynecology under the title "Maternal Deaths Associated with an Intrauterine Device." The American Journal of Obstetrics & Gynecology was, ironically, the same journal that four years earlier had published the Hugh Davis article that gave the Shield its original respectability.

Christian's tone throughout the article stressed the urgency and deadly seriousness of his report.

"It is the purpose of this communication to report two maternal deaths and make reference to three others (as well as several severely septic midtrimester abortions) in which a pattern of pathophysiology is surfacing that appears to be associated more commonly with a particular intra-uterine device," Christian reported. "These cases are being referred to rather than completely detailed because of a sense of urgency to express the author's concern regarding the possible problems with [the Dalkon Shield]."

Christian wrote that he was particularly concerned with "the rather insidious yet rapid manner in which these patients became ill. In three of the five noted maternal deaths, the first symptoms, which were disarm-ingly innocuous in and of themselves, occurred within 31 to 71 hours of death."

Christian said he wasn't sure exactly what it was about the Shield that had led to these infections, although he speculated that it had something to do with the device's shape. His article did not implicate the tail string in the infections; but, then, Christian did not know at that time, as A. H. Robins did, that the tail string wicked.

Although he acknowledged that the Centers for Disease Control had recently sent out a questionnaire to doctors about IUD-related deaths and hospitalizations, Christian had some harsh words for the government's ineffectiveness in evaluating and controlling medical devices like the Shield. "Certainly, if there were five botulism deaths from one type of mushroom soup, the Food and Drug Administration would do more than put out a questionnaire," he wrote.

A. H. Robins officials, of course, had known the article was coming. In May, the company had anticipated the article by sending a "Dear Doctor" letter to 120,000 obstetricians, gynecologists, internists, family practitioners, and osteopaths around the country. This letter essentially passed on the recommendations of the doctors who had attended the company's septic abortion conference: Every patient who misses a men-strual period while wearing the Dalkon Shield should have a pregnancy test. As soon as a pregnancy is confirmed, the Shield should be removed. If it can't be removed easily, "serious consideration should be given to offering the patient a therapeutic abortion." If a woman opts to continue her pregnancy, she should be followed very closely for early signs of sepsis.

A. H. Robins knew the letter would have a detrimental effect on sales of the Shield—but how detrimental was still a matter of debate. The medical staff was more optimistic about the Shield's chances of withstanding yet another round of bad publicity than the marketing staff. But then, the marketing staff had been staring at the Shield's slumping sales figures for many months. According to a status report dated May 24, 1974, sales of the Shield were down 31 percent from May of the previous year. And through April 1974, sales were even more miserable, running 48.3 percent behind a comparable 1973 period. The only bright spot in the sales picture was the overseas market, where sales of the Shield were climbing. But with the issuance of the "Dear Doctor" letter, A. H. Robins' marketing experts believed that international sales would follow the downward trend seen domestically.

The future looked gloomy for the Shield. Inside the company, there was talk about taking the device off the market. But there was the troubling problem of lawsuits. By the end of May 1974, 47 suits by users of the Dalkon Shield had been filed, asking for damages totaling in excess of $25 million. A. H. Robins' attorney Roger Tuttle opposed a recall of the device, arguing that such a recall would harm the company's position in court. "It is the opinion of Mr. Tuttle that if this product is taken off the market it will be a 'confession of liability' and Robins would lose many of the pending lawsuits," said the May 1974 progress report.

Tuttle predicted that a lengthy legal battle lay ahead for A. H. Robins. "The point was made that whether this product were taken off the market or allowed to die slowly, there would still be lawsuits 'in process' for as long as 10 years in the future," the progress report noted. (When this prediction was read back to him 10 years later in a Minnesota courtroom, Tuttle wryly commented that "My accuracy approaches a hundred percent in this case.")

Nowhere in that progress report was there a discussion of the long battle women would have to fight in their personal lives if the Shield were not recalled, but allowed instead to "die slowly" in their wombs. The health—indeed, the lives—of millions of women did not merit consideration in this "progress report."

Soon after A. H. Robins sent its "Dear Doctor" letters out, the worst fears of the company's marketing department came true. On May 28, 1974, the Planned Parenthood Federation instructed its 183 clinics to stop prescribing the Dalkon Shield immediately because of the threat of sepsis. "It is imperative that we act with all appropriate caution to safeguard the interest of our patients," said a Planned Parenthood spokesperson. Planned Parenthood officials also expressed their anger at A. H. Robins for not notifying them directly about the sepsis problem. Although many of their 89,000 IUD users had been fitted with Dalkon Shields, Planned Parenthood officials said they had only learned about the "Dear Doctor" letter and its contents accidentally from private physicians. A. H. Robins officials agree in retrospect that this was a regrettable oversight on their part.

Other clinics soon followed Planned Parenthood's lead. Health officials in Maryland and Virginia—home states for Hugh Davis and the A. H. Robins Company—directed their state clinic doctors to stop prescribing the Dalkon Shield. Both states reported that the Shield had been widely used in their clinics; Maryland officials estimated that the Shield made up 61 percent of state-prescribed IUDs.

On June 11, 1974, Fred Clark went before an FDA Ob-Gyn Medical Devices Panel to present A. H. Robins' case for the Shield. The panel was part of the Bureau of Medical Devices and was looking into the septic abortion problem. A similar panel, working under the FDA's Bureau of Drugs, was also studying the problem. In an impassioned speech to the device panel, Clark argued that the Shield should not be singled out among IUDs for causing septic abortions. As A. H. Robins officials had done before, and would do again, Clark hinted that at least some of the blame for problems with the Shield rested with doctors (improper insertion of the device) or with women (self-induced abortions). He acknowledged that the very nature of an IUD—the way it causes an inflammatory reaction in the uterus—might play a role in infection, but that this factor was certainly not unique to the Dalkon Shield. Of course, what was unique to the Dalkon Shield was its multifilament string. But Clark did not pass that bit of information on to the FDA panel.

On June 24, members of the FDA's Medical Devices Panel issued a draft report asking A. H. Robins to stop sales of the Shield and recall devices already sold "because of the health hazard." If A. H. Robins didn't go along with the recommendation, the report said, the FDA should seize the Shield as it had done with the Majzlin Spring. On June 26, 1974, FDA Commissioner Alexander Schmidt wrote a letter to E. Claiborne Robins, Sr., requesting that A. H. Robins stop marketing the Dalkon Shield until its "questionable safety" could be reviewed by the agency. Two days later, the company complied.

Although Schmidt's request to suspend sales was bad news for A. H. Robins, the FDA commissioner did not follow the Medical Devices Panel's recommendation that he ask the company to recall the Shield. That was considered a small victory at A. H. Robins headquarters, where, on July 2, 1974, Chairman E. Claiborne Robins, Sr., wrote a memo telling some of his staff that they had "performed a seemingly impossible task" in containing the FDA actions to a suspension of sales. "We had all felt that the decision would be political, and to have Dr.

Schmidt announce his action—taken against the vote of the [advisory] panels—was indicative of the input of our team which had been working constantly with the FDA during the period leading up to the announcement."

Indeed, the mild tone of the FDA's press release announcing that A. H. Robins had decided to suspend sales of the Shield—a press release company officials had helped draft—"helped reinforce our image as an ethical pharmaceutical company, which places the safety and efficacy of our products in a primary position," E. Claiborne Robins, Sr., added in his memo.

The rest of the summer brought only more bad news for A. H. Robins. In July, the Centers for Disease Control in Atlanta publicly reported the findings of its survey of 34,544 physicians throughout the country about their experience with IUDs. The findings indicated that fatal septic abortions occurred twice as frequently among Shield users as among women who wore other IUDs. (A. H. Robins claims the survey was deficient because of flaws in its methodology and because only half the doctors who were sent questionnaires responded.)

By the end of August 1974, the FDA had reports that 11 women had died and other 209 had become seriously ill from septic abortions while wearing the Dalkon Shield. This compared to reports of five deaths and 21 septic illnesses among Lippes Loop wearers (which had been on the market much longer than the Shield) and one death and eight septic illnesses among Saf-T-Coil users.

The public was now clamoring for some answers. To decide once and for all whether or not the Shield was more dangerous than other IUDs, the FDA convened a special panel, charged with coming to some conclusions about the safety and efficacy of the Shield; the panel was made up of the members of the existing Drug and Device panels. The major question to be answered, of course, was: Is the Shield more likely than other IUDs to cause septic abortions?

The FDA sent A. H. Robins written requests for information regarding the Dalkon Shield's safety and efficacy. Among the specific questions for which the FDA wanted answers were those dealing with the testing of the Shield: What studies had been conducted? Was the device changed as a result of those studies? Were any deaths or injuries reported in those studies? Upon what evidence did A. H. Robins rely in claiming that its product was safe and effective and could be commercially marketed? The FDA also asked A. H. Robins to produce copies of any available reports, studies, or correspondence dealing with the experience of doctors, clinics, or hospitals that had been using the Shield.

A. H. Robins' response to this part of the FDA request for information was "This information will be supplied at a later date."

On August 15, 1974, a memo from A. H. Robins' President William Zimmer asked 15 A. H. Robins officials to search their files "for *any* letters, memos or notes on oral or written communications relating in any way to the thread utilized for the tail for the Dalkon Shield. . . . Of particular interest are any references to 'wicking' of the tail. To the extent that you have had any oral communications with third parties on this subject which are not memorialized in writing, please submit a memo on any such communication. . . . This project is of utmost importance, and should be completed by Friday, August 16."

As a result of this request, Ken Moore, the Shield's project manager, wrote two chronologies detailing the correspondence and other activities of A. H. Robins officials regarding the Shield's tail string. Although these chronologies mention references in the correspondence to wicking being a problem, none of the letters or memos or even the concerns expressed in the correspondence were forwarded to the FDA. Some of these letters and memos have since disappeared from A. H. Robins' files.

On August 21 and 22, the FDA Drug and Device panels were combined into one 18-member panel that became known as the Ad Hoc Committee and held 13 hours of public hearings on the Shield. Thirty-two people testified before the panel, and the testimony was often conflicting. Donald Christian spoke out harshly against the Shield, pointing out that reports of spontaneous septic abortions in the second trimester of pregnancy had been almost unheard of before. "This is a new phenomenon," he told the panel. "In my simple way I have to conclude that maybe it's associated [predominantly with the Shield]."

Daniel Mishall, a gynecologist at the University of Southern California, concurred. He presented data showing that with the use of the Shield, perforation of the uterus occurred more frequently and with more serious complications than with other devices.

But then along came Robert Snowden, a sociologist at the University of Exeter in England, in support of the Shield. "The crude perforation rate associated with the Dalkon Shield is much lower than that for the Lippes Loop," he said.

Fred Clark was also there, claiming, again, that any condemnation of the Shield was totally unjustified. He argued that the Dalkon Shield was no less safe than other IUDs—it had only received more publicity and thus more adverse reports.

But the presentation that seemed to make the most impression on the panel came from Howard Tatum. Although his study would not be published for another six months, Tatum outlined for the panel what he had found out about the Shield's tail string. It could harbor and wick bacteria into the uterus. And in a pregnant woman, the entire bacteria-laden tail string could be pulled into the uterus as the fetus grew.

A decade later, A. H. Robins still complains about Tatum and his study. According to Fletcher Owen, A. H. Robins' director of medical services, "Tatum has his own reasons for making things look bad for the Dalkon Shield." Owen points out that Tatum has "devoted his life to IUDs" and hints that Tatum wanted in 1974 to make the Shield look bad so all IUDs, including his own "T" device, wouldn't be blacklisted. There are some acknowledged flaws in Tatum's study. Most notably, by coating the tail strings in petroleum jelly, Tatum may have ruled out the possibility that bacteria travels up the "outside" of monofilament strings as well as the "inside" of the Shield's multifilament one. Indeed, the FDA believes this may very well happen—but only after years of wear. It takes that long, says the FDA, for protein deposits, which apparently provide a foothold for bacteria, to build up on the outside of monofilament strings. Those flaws in Tatum's study, however, have nothing to do with the validity of his findings on the Dalkon Shield.

After listening to two days of testimony, the Ad Hoc Committee concluded that IUDs in general were relatively safe and effective. The Dalkon Shield, however, seemed to be causing more serious problems in women than the other IUDs and the Ad Hoc Committee thought a special review was needed.

But the Ad Hoc Committee members were anything but unanimous in their concerns about the safety of the Dalkon Shield. After the August 21 and 22 hearings concluded, members of the Device Panel who had served on the Ad Hoc Committee met for lunch and agreed that the moratorium on sales of the Shield should continue. A short time later, the members of the Device Panel met in a closed session with the Ad Hoc Committee members from the Drug Panel.

The mere fact that Drug Panel members were included in the process bothered Dr. Richard Dickey, an associate professor of obstetrics and gynecology at the Louisiana State University School of Medicine in New Orleans and a member of the Device Panel. "One can raise at this point a legitimate question about why the . . . Drug Panel was included [in the decision making], since the Dalkon Shield is a device and not a drug," Dickey later told a congressional committee looking into the FDA's handling of the Shield.

Unable to reach a decision on whether the moratorium on Shield sales should be continued, the Ad Hoc Committee formed a subcommittee to try to resolve the problem. The subcommittee was made up of four members from the Drug Panel and four members from the Device Panel.

The subcommittee met on Labor Day weekend, when two members who had originally supported continuing the moratorium could not attend. The subcommittee drafted a report that read, "It is not apparent that the safety and efficacy of the Dalkon Shield is significantly different from other IUDs." After the draft report was circulated to all 18 members of the Ad Hoc Committee, a telephone vote was taken and the panel accepted the report by a 12-to-6 margin.

The FDA was prepared to announce that the Shield could go back on the market, under strict supervision, and that announcement was timed for the final meeting of the Ad Hoc Committee in October 1974. At that meeting, however, members who originally opposed allowing the Shield back on the market requested that safety questions about the device be reopened for debate.

Several members said they had not understood when they voted for the subcommittee's draft report that it amounted to an endorsement of allowing the Shield back on the market, and they now wanted to change their votes. A new vote was taken, and the meeting ended with the Ad Hoc Committee changing its recommendation from lifting the ban on the Shield to stating that "the moratorium on commercial distribution of the Dalkon Shield remain in effect pending accumulation of definitive data."

"That this was not the expected result [by the FDA] was evident from the fact that [FDA Commissioner Alexander Schmidt] canceled his press conference scheduled for that afternoon," Dickey said later, "and did not announce his decision for action until December 20, nearly two months later."

When Schmidt finally made his December 20 announcement, his decision stunned Dickey and other panel members. Without telling any of the panel members in advance, Schmidt announced in a press conference that sale of the Shield would be resumed—just the opposite of the Ad Hoc Committee's final recommendation. The restriction Schmidt placed on the remarketing of the Shield was that a tight registry system would be put in place.

The new registry system, to be run by A. H. Robins, would require that each new Dalkon Shield be numbered and tracked. Doctors who wanted to participate in the program would keep track of the women they inserted with the Shield and report back to A. H. Robins on any problems. Only doctors who agreed to follow this procedure would be allowed to insert the new Dalkon Shields. A. H. Robins was to maintain a computer file of the new insertions and follow-up reports and tabulate the figures quarterly. The results were to be passed on to the FDA every six months.

Dickey said the registry program was "of very dubious scientific value" and had not been approved by the combined panel.

Three days after Schmidt's announcement, Dr. Emanuel Friedman of Boston's Beth Israel Hospital, resigned from the Device Panel and the combined panel and urged other members to join him. In a letter to Horace Thompson, chairman of the Device Panel, Friedman wrote: "I feel my effectiveness as a member of the panel is at an end. Moreover, I do not feel that the advisory committee, consisting of both the drug and device panels, has had any impact whatsoever on the activities of the Food and Drug Administration relative to its recent action terminating the moratorium on use of the Dalkon Shield."

Schmidt had told the press, Friedman wrote, that the FDA action "did not constitute an overruling of the committee's recommendation. [T]hat is clearly not the case." Ultimately, the Ad Hoc Committee had "almost unanimously" recommended the Shield stay off the market, Friedman said. "I would urge other members of the emasculated panel to join with me in this protest action, thereby lending collective support to the contention that Doctor Schmidt acted inappropriately."

None of the other panel members resigned, and several said they didn't think what Schmidt did was wrong.

The registry system never got off the drawing boards, however—and the Dalkon Shield never went back on the market.

Lillian Yin, now head of the FDA's division of Ob-Gyn Medical Devices, was working with the advisory panels after Schmidt announced plans for the registry system. An epidemiology study done after the announcement indicated the registry system "would never have worked," she said. It would have been too difficult to try to keep track of the women who received new Shields, she said.

Yin, however, thought Friedman and Dickey overreacted to Schmidt's announcement of the registry system. "You announce a program like that to let people comment on it," she said. The FDA, Yin said, also insisted that A. H. Robins do a detailed study of the Shield (information gathered from the registry system was a significant part of that study), even if the company decided to bring the device back with a monofilament tail string. On November 12, 1974, with the FDA panels clearly against lifting the Shield moratorium, A. H. Robins had sent the agency a telegram notifying it of the company's decision to change the multifilament tail string to a monofilament tail string and reintroduce the Shield.

On December 6, in a meeting with A. H. Robins, FDA officials made it clear that, while they thought the monofilament string was a good idea, "under no circumstances would the FDA agree to uncontrolled distribution of the Dalkon Shield." "At the time we weren't sure if it was the tail string or the design [that was causing the infections in women]," Yin said. The FDA wanted the device tested, no matter how it was changed.

A. H. Robins delayed a decision on the Shield for several months. Finally, on August 8, 1975, citing the ongoing bad publicity the Shield was receiving, A. H. Robins announced that it had abandoned all plans to remarket the device.

A. H. Robins also said it remained firm in its belief that the Dalkon Shield, when properly used, was a safe and effective device.

The Shield was finally, and permanently, off the market—at least in the United States. But it was still in the bodies of hundreds of thousands of unsuspecting women.

A year later, in 1976, the FDA got what it wanted from Congress— the tougher medical device legislation it had so sorely needed six years earlier. The legislation, in the form of amendments to the 1938 Food, Drug, and Cosmetic Act, gave the agency the power to require device manufacturers to prove their products were safe before putting them on the market.

If such a law had been on the books in 1970, the story of the Dalkon Shield might have been much different.

Cynthia

"Every time I have a baby, I say, 'Okay, I have one more. But I'm missing one.'"

—Cynthia Parker

*I*n the fall of 1972, Cynthia Parker, a 24-year-old flight attendant for Northwest Airlines, went to see her doctor in Bloomington, Minnesota, about some burning and itching she was experiencing in her vagina. The doctor diagnosed the problem as a yeast infection, a very common and uncomfortable, but not serious, infection experienced by women during their menstrual years.

During her exam, Cynthia asked her doctor about birth control. She had been taking the Pill for a short period of time, but believed it was making her nauseous. And she didn't like the idea of taking hormones that might be altering the chemistry of her body.

The doctor suggested an IUD. Cynthia had read a little about these devices. She knew they were put inside the uterus to create an environment that would inhibit contraception. But that was about all she knew.

Her doctor pulled an IUD out of a drawer. Small and white with round feet-like appendages, the device reminded Cynthia of a spider. It was, of course, the Dalkon Shield.

Her doctor said the Shield would be the best IUD for her because it came in two sizes. The smaller size was made especially for women who had never had children, and the doctor told Cynthia her body would be less likely to reject it.

A couple of months later, after her yeast infection had cleared up,

Cynthia returned to the clinic to be fitted with a Dalkon Shield. The insertion was extremely painful; she almost fainted. She experienced additional pain for two more days, but eventually it went away and she forgot about the device within her uterus.

In July, Cynthia married Terry, a former U.S. Army Military Intelligence sergeant who had recently begun working for his father's construction company in Minneapolis. After the wedding, which was held in the small Iowa town of Naushau, Cynthia and Terry flew to the Fiji Islands and Hawaii for their honeymoon.

Although Cynthia and Terry both loved children, they had decided to put off having their own for a while. Terry had been married before and had recently been given custody of his four-year-old son, Jon. Both Cynthia and Terry believed it was important for them and Jon to get acquainted before adding any other members to the family. Cynthia figured the IUD would protect her from pregnancy.

Shortly after returning to Minneapolis from her honeymoon, Cynthia had what she thought was a very light menstrual period. Then she began to feel nauseous, especially around the cigarette smoke of Northwest's passengers. Her co-workers began to tease her about being pregnant. *I can't be*, Cynthia told herself, *I'm wearing an IUD.*

But as the days passed, the symptoms of pregnancy became more pronounced. Cynthia found it difficult to sustain her energy level while working, and during flight layovers in other cities, she would sleep for 12 hours at a time.

In August 1973, Cynthia went back to her doctor for a pregnancy test. It was positive. Although she had not wanted to become pregnant quite this soon, Cynthia was still ecstatic about the idea of becoming a mother. "I remember going out of the doctor's office on a cloud," she recalls.

The doctor had told her that he could not remove the Dalkon Shield from her uterus because the procedure might cause a miscarriage. He reassured her, however, that by leaving the device in, her chances of miscarriage were only 10 percent greater than those of a woman without the device.

When Cynthia asked about whether the device could pierce and damage her child's body, the doctor was also calming. He drew a picture for her of how the baby would be protected from the device by the placenta. Nothing to worry about, he reassured her.

As it turned out, however, Cynthia had a lot to worry about. Only a couple of weeks after that first exam, while preparing her family's dinner, Cynthia felt a sudden pain in her abdomen. It was so strong and persistent she couldn't stand, and she had to lie down on the couch, her knees drawn toward her chest. Terry took her to the doctor. They were both afraid she would lose the baby.

After examining Cynthia, the doctor told her the pain she was experiencing was her uterus contracting as it attempted to expel the IUD. He told her again not to worry. He also noted in his conversation with her that he could no longer feel the Shield's tail string in her vagina. It had been drawn up into her uterus.

About a week after this exam, Cynthia began to notice a brown discharge from her vagina. She called her doctor. Again he told her it was nothing serious. The discharge, he said rather cryptically, was simply "old blood."

The painful contractions and brownish discharge continued into Cynthia's fourth month of pregnancy. Finally, Cynthia's doctor gave her some medicine to relax her uterus and stop the bleeding and contractions. He told her he wanted her to come back in two days for another pregnancy test to make sure she had not, perhaps, spontaneously aborted the baby earlier.

Cynthia drove home. By the time she reached her home she was bleeding profusely. She couldn't move without passing large clots of blood from her vagina. The heavy bleeding continued into the night.

By morning, the bleeding had turned into spotting and the cramping had stopped. The drug had apparently done its job. Nor had Cynthia lost the baby. When she went for a pregnancy test the next day, the result was again positive.

For the next few weeks, everything went well. Cynthia began to feel the baby's soft butterfly-like movements within her. She and Terry started shopping for a house in Minneapolis' suburbs, and Cynthia began to embroider a baby's blanket.

At her five-month exam, Cynthia heard the baby's heartbeat for the first time. Her doctor used an amplified stethoscope and the quick rhythmic thumps of the baby's heart echoed through the examining room. Cynthia was very excited.

The following day, she woke up with a fever. By mid-morning she was experiencing some slight cramping and the spotting of blood also returned. She called her doctor. He told her to call him back if any watery fluid leaked from her vagina or if her temperature rose.

Around ten o'clock, Cynthia's water broke and the fever was so bad that she was shaking uncontrollably. She called the doctor again. He told her to come to his office immediately.

Cynthia had a friend drive her to the clinic. The doctor listened to the baby's heartbeat; he told her that it had changed from the day before and was now beating abnormally. "I'm putting you in the hospital," he said.

At that point, the nightmare really began for Cynthia. At the hospital she was put through a series of tests. She was told she had an infection of some kind, but the doctors weren't clear about its cause.

Finally, she was told that the infection was in her uterus and that it had triggered labor. Her baby was on its way—four months too soon. Any attempt to try to stop the baby's delivery would surely kill Cynthia, for the infection could not then be successfully treated and it would only grow worse and spread through her bloodstream. No one came right out and told Cynthia that the baby would surely die soon after birth, if it wasn't dead already. But she knew.

Cynthia was experiencing a spontaneous septic abortion in the second trimester of her pregnancy—a very rare and life-threatening condition.

The doctors did not give Cynthia a reason for the infection and she was too sick to ask for one. She gave them permission to administer a drug to hurry along the labor that had already begun. She was told she would have to go through a "normal" labor and delivery, just as if she were delivering a full-term baby.

Terry was called and he quickly drove to the hospital. He was terrified that Cynthia might die. He stayed with Cynthia throughout her labor; a long, hard labor that lasted well into the night.

Cynthia cried through most of it. She knew she would be delivering a dead baby. At one point, when the contractions were at their peak, she screamed with despair at the nurses and doctors around her; "Let's get this over with because I'm not getting anything out of it anyway."

Sometime after midnight, the baby was delivered. Terry had been told to leave the delivery room a short time before.

"I said, 'Here it comes,' " Cynthia recalls. "I could feel it go through the birth canal." The child was so small, it simply slipped through the canal without any of the usual struggle and trauma of delivery.

"Oh, it's a girl," the doctor said as the baby emerged from Cynthia's body. The tone of his voice was light, as if he were passing on some joyful information to the mother of a live and fully developed, newborn baby. It may have been an instinctive reaction on the doctor's part, but the words hurt Cynthia deeply.

"I want to see it," Cynthia told him.

"No you don't," the doctor responded.

"Yes, I do," Cynthia insisted.

She pulled herself up on her elbows to look at her tiny daughter.

Lifting the baby up by the feet, the doctor held her in front of Cynthia.

"Here it is," he said.

The baby was tiny and perfectly formed—and burgundy red in color. Cynthia was told later that the reddishness was due to the fact that the baby's final layer of skin had not yet formed.

Cynthia never got a chance to touch or hold the baby, for the doctor immediately removed the child from the delivery room. "He just walked out with what he felt was a blob," Cynthia recalls. "That was my baby. I don't even know where the baby went."

As the doctor was leaving, Cynthia heard him say, "Oh, the IUD." A few moments later he returned to retrieve the device. He found it wrapped in the placenta.

Cynthia spent several days in the hospital recovering from the birth and from the infection. Antibiotics finally made her well again. But only physically. Emotionally, she had a difficult time ahead.

"I remember crying for months," Cynthia recalls. She became determined to get pregnant again, and slightly more than a year later delivered a healthy, full-term baby girl, whom she named Kari. Three more children followed: Mollie, Abbi, and Evan.

"I've had four babies since," Cynthia acknowledges, "but after each birth I couldn't help but remember that first baby. My husband and I didn't name her. But Mollie did a couple of years ago. She calls her Sara. Last Mother's Day all the kids made me a card and signed it. They put Sara's name on it, too."

15

First Trial

"[The doctor] said she wouldn't use one of those things in a dog."

—Bradley Post, plaintiffs' attorney.

When Connie Deemer walked into his Wichita law office in 1972, Bradley Post had no idea that her case would change not only the direction of Dalkon Shield litigation, but the course of his own professional life.

At that time, Post was a 42-year-old products liability and medical negligence attorney. Soft-spoken, low-keyed, with a dark serious face that resembled that of television newscaster Sam Donaldson, Post had a small, but reputable Wichita practice in 1972. He wasn't looking for a cause. Yet within a few years, Post would find himself at the center of the Dalkon Shield litigation. And the eye of this legal storm, unlike that of a hurricane, would be anything but calm.

On that day in 1972, however, when Post first interviewed Connie Deemer, nothing about the case seemed particularly out of the ordinary. On August 10, 1971, Connie's obstetrician had inserted a small plastic IUD into her uterus. The doctor told her that the device was as effective as the birth control pill, but that it wouldn't cause cancer.

Only two months before the insertion, Connie had given birth to her first child, a girl. She hadn't wanted to become pregnant again, at least not right away.

The insertion was extremely painful for Connie—worse than labor, she said—and the pain continued for two days. When it finally subsided,

Connie settled down to taking care of her infant daughter, confident that at least she wouldn't have to worry about birth control.

But the IUD failed and two months later Connie became pregnant again. During the exam that confirmed her pregnancy, Connie's doctor couldn't feel the Shield's tail string in Connie's vagina. It had either slipped out unnoticed by Connie or had been pulled into her uterus. If it was in the uterus, her doctor said, removing it could be very dangerous for the baby.

Although Connie had not wanted to become pregnant so soon, an abortion was out of the question for her, for she did not believe in them. She continued the pregnancy, terrified that the device might cause her to miscarry or that it might somehow lodge itself in her unborn baby's brain—a fear about IUDs she had picked up from talking with other women.

Fortunately, the Dalkon Shield didn't cause Connie to go into premature labor as it had so many other women, and on June 22, 1972, after carrying her second child to full term, she gave birth to another girl. It was less than one year after the birth of her first. Connie was relieved to discover that the device had not pierced her child's head, but neither could it be found in Connie's uterus.

Connie's doctor assumed the IUD had been expelled before Connie became pregnant, but just to make sure, she had Connie X-rayed at her first postpartum examination. To everyone's surprise, the Shield showed up in the X-ray; it had perforated Connie's uterus and lodged itself in her abdominal cavity near her appendix.

Doctors surgically removed the IUD, leaving Connie with a permanent scar on her abdomen. The surgery left her unable to care for her two young daughters for several weeks. It also left Connie angry. She had been told that her chances of getting pregnant while wearing this IUD were very slim—around one percent. And she had not been told that the device could perforate her uterus.

Connie contacted an attorney, who, in turn, referred her to Post. Post was then with the law firm of Michaud and Cranmer, a firm with a growing reputation for representing plaintiffs in medical negligence and drug products liability cases.

When she first spoke with Post, Connie didn't even know which kind of IUD had caused her problem. But to Post it didn't matter. He expected to sue the doctor who had inserted the device, not the company that made it. This was, he told Connie, a clear-cut case of medical malpractice, of a doctor who had erred. Post agreed to take on the case for a standard contingency fee. In other words, if Connie won the case or settled it out of court, Post would get a percentage of the amount won or settled. If the case was lost, Connie would pay Post nothing.

Within weeks, Post deposed—took testimony under oath from—Connie's doctor, who revealed that the device she had inserted into Connie's uterus was the Dalkon Shield. The doctor said she had begun recommending the Shield to her patients after a visit to her office by a detailman from A. H. Robins. The detailman had shown the doctor a movie about the Shield—the one produced by Win Lerner and Thad Earl in Earl's Defiance office—and had given her an impressive-looking, published medical article. Both the movie and the article professed that the device had a 1.1 percent pregnancy rate and was a "superior" IUD.

Post next talked to the detailman, who confirmed that he had represented the Shield to Connie's doctor as a "superior" device. And he had a scientific paper to prove it, a paper written by a well-known doctor at Johns Hopkins: Dr. Hugh Davis. Post read the paper, and noted that Davis wrote of having wonderful success with the device.

So, it seemed that Post's initial reaction had been right: Connie's complaint was with her doctor and with her doctor only. A simple case of medical malpractice. After all, there was no evidence pointing in the direction of A. H. Robins, no reason not to believe their claims that the Dalkon Shield was a superior IUD. And they had the impressive-looking study from Johns Hopkins to back up those claims. It seemed, on the surface at least, that Connie's doctor had simply botched up the insertion.

But under the surface, something about the case was troubling Post. Within six months of taking on Connie Deemer's case, three other Dalkon Shield cases were referred to him. All three cases, like Connie's, involved perforation of the uterus, yet each woman had had a different doctor. Was it a coincidence that four doctors had been negligent with the same device? Or was it more reasonable to assume that it was the device that was at fault?

And why had he suddenly come upon four Dalkon Shield cases when he had seen only two or three other IUD cases within the previous six years? Was there something particularly menacing about the Dalkon Shield? Post wanted to find out, so he decided to sue A. H. Robins as well as Connie's doctor for Connie's injuries.

What Post didn't know was that other attorneys across the country were also growing suspicious of the Shield and filing suits against A. H. Robins. In the spring of 1972, only a trickle of claims was coming into the legal offices at A. H. Robins; soon it would turn into a deluge.

The pretrial discovery process began innocently enough. This is the process through which both parties in a lawsuit gather facts and information from each other to help prepare for trial. Post flew out to Richmond to look through thousands of A. H. Robins' documents. It was a tiring procedure. Each document had to be read thoroughly and marked. Post knew what he was looking for: any document that might show that the Dalkon Shield was not all what it was claimed to be. But he also knew that finding such a document would be like finding a needle in a haystack.

A. H. Robins' lead attorney for the Dalkon Shield cases was Roger Tuttle, who, unbeknownst to Post, was having a very difficult time getting the cooperation of A. H. Robins' medical department in his efforts to defend the Shield. As A. H. Robins' in-house attorney, Tuttle had dealt with a few other claims against the Shield, but Post was the first to demand document production. It was, Tuttle recalled later, a major undertaking. "He asked for every piece of paper we had," Tuttle said.

When Tuttle received Post's request for the Shield documents he went to court in an unsuccessful attempt to limit it as much as possible. At the same time Tuttle told Fletcher Owen of A. H. Robins' medical department that, "You got a job nights, weekends, holidays, whatever. This has got to be done." Fred Clark, Owen's boss, complained bitterly about the document request because compliance was going to require considerable overtime work for the medical department. Tuttle told him it didn't matter; there was a court order and the work had to be done.

Documents were gathered but Tuttle ran into what he later described as "a Chinese wall." "The mandate to me was to defend the litigation," Tuttle testified a decade later. "I got grudging cooperation at best. In many instances I got no cooperation at all. I was constantly surprised by the A. H. Robins medical department because they were forever pulling rabbits out of the hat that I didn't think existed."

One of those rabbits was Fred Clark's memo of June 9, 1970, the memo in which Clark points out that the data used by Hugh Davis in his 1970 paper was invalid. This, of course, meant that the company knew that Davis' 12-month study, the basis of all their "superior" claims, was invalid.

The damning document itself, containing what Tuttle called a "devastating admission," was dumped almost literally in Post's lap.

The day of the document production, Post, Tuttle, Owen, Ken Moore, and a host of others were gathered around a table in a meeting room in A. H. Robins' medical department. The documents were brought in, and Tuttle, working with Wichita attorney Robert Siefkin, who had been hired by A. H. Robins to work with Tuttle on the Deemer case, tried to review them before handing them to Post. Tuttle looked

163

through one box of documents while Siefkin checked another. When Tuttle or Siefkin came across a document that they believed was legally privileged—not subject to disclosure in a court of law because of some special circumstance, such as a communication between a client and attorney—they would put it aside. In his later testimony, Tuttle recounted the key moment in the document production—a moment that changed the course of all future litigation.

"It was toward the end of the review by the various attorneys, and I believe Post said, 'Well is this everything?' and I said yes, it was. But I said, 'Let me check and make certain.'

"And I went to Owen and I said, 'Do we have everything?' And I believe his initial response was yes, and I went back in the room and very shortly thereafter someone brought [another file] and said, 'Well, we found this additional material,' and simply unceremoniously dumped it on the table. And the fat was in the fire."

The documents from the file, Tuttle said, "were dumped physically so that Mr. Post got his hands on them first. And again, rather than have a wrestling match between gentlemen, we all were sitting around this table and, as a consequence they were circulated."

Tuttle was sitting next to Post when Post reached into the pile of documents and pulled out the Clark memo on the pregnancy rate. "In a sense, he and I stumbled onto the thing almost simultaneously," Tuttle said, "but he had physical possession of it. And, at that point in time, of course, it was too late to do anything about it."

Post, of course, was astonished to find such a document laying on the table in front of him. He could only give it a cursory read at that time, however, for he wasn't sure if Tuttle and the other lawyers present realized the importance of the memo and he did not want to tip them off. But he knew that with that memo the Connie Deemer case was off and running.

Tuttle, on the other hand, knew that, with the exposure of the memo, A. H. Robins was in serious trouble. Tuttle later said that he was "chagrined and embarrassed" by Post's discovery of the memo "because the counsel for the other side in important litigation had come upon a document which I felt my client should have provided me with before it was simply made available to the other side."

But the incident was even more disturbing to Tuttle for another reason. As he read the Clark memo for the first time it became "self-evident" to Tuttle that Hugh Davis, in his original clinical testing of the Shield—the testing upon which the Shield was being promoted—had used a "method of opting in and opting out of his studies women who . . .

showed good results in the use of the Shield as opposed to those that didn't."

"In point of fact, what Clark is saying to me in this paper is that his investigation would cause a knowledgeable pharmaceutical house to raise serious questions about the validity of Davis' study if he was in effect playing the numbers game, taking the good results and saying that's one study and publishing on that, and at the same time opting out the bad results and in a sense burying those. It would make the device appear to perform better than in fact it did."

After the discovery process session in which Post pulled the incriminating Clark memo from the pile, Tuttle went to Clark and "hit the ceiling." When he tried to impress upon Clark just how damaging the memo would be to the Deemer litigation, Clark showed little, if any, concern, Tuttle said.

"I kind of felt like he patted me on the head and said 'Go defend the lawsuits and don't bother me . . . until you have important matters,' " Tuttle said.

The memo, as Tuttle anticipated, became the cornerstone of Connie Deemer's case. Post dubbed it "the secret memorandum." It was the first loose thread found in the tightly woven fabric of A. H. Robins' Dalkon Shield defense.

Connie Deemer's case went to trial in Wichita in December of 1974. It was the second Dalkon Shield case to be argued in court, and the first to be completed. Another Shield case in California had ended in a mistrial only a few weeks earlier.

Post had actually hoped one of his other Dalkon Shield cases would be tried first, for he felt it was a stronger case to take to a jury. The woman in that case had suffered more serious injuries than Connie; for the Shield, after perforating her uterus, had also nicked her colon, causing an infection. She underwent a temporary colostomy to divert undigested food from the inflamed part of her colon.

But Connie's case had been filed first, and Post was unsuccessful in his legal maneuverings to get it pushed back on the court's calendar. In her suit, Connie asked for $70,000 in compensatory damages from both her doctor and A. H. Robins, and $250,000 in punitive damages. Compensatory damages are meant to compensate an injured party for the injury he or she sustained. Punitive damages are awarded over and above the injury sustained. As the term implies, punitive damages are meant to punish the party that caused the injury.

In his one-and-a-half-hour opening statement, Post outlined his evidence for the jury of six women and six men. Like other pharmaceutical companies, Post said, A. H. Robins had taken advantage of the Pill scare to promote an IUD—in this case, the Dalkon Shield. Its labeling and advertisements claimed the device to be safe and effective, yet the company had not adequately tested the device to back up those claims. Indeed, when it learned that the pregnancy rate for the Shield was actually higher than the initial study had indicated, it chose to suppress those facts rather than change its advertising claims.

Post also charged the company with not publicizing its knowledge that "the device has side effects, side effects that can kill." One of those side effects, he said, was the complication experienced by Connie Deemer: perforation of the uterus. The company was "grossly and wantonly negligent," Post concluded, for disregarding the harm its product would cause to the women who wore it. In other words, Connie was entitled to punitive as well as compensatory damages.

When Post sat down after his opening statement, Robert Siefkin rose to present A. H. Robins' side to the jury. The evidence will show that the Dalkon Shield is no more dangerous than other types of devices, Siefkin told the jury, and although some doctors have had trouble with the device, many, many others have not, as the jury would soon hear.

Connie's difficulty with the Shield, Siefkin continued, was the result of her own anatomy: She had a retroverted uterus, and A. H. Robins had clearly warned doctors not to insert the Shield in the one-quarter of the American female population who have this "abnormal" condition. Her doctor should have heeded this warning, Siefkin indicated.

And so the stage was set for a dramatic courtroom battle. The trial ran for two months. Russel Thomsen, the Army major who had earlier blasted the Shield before Congress, testified, relating his belief that the Shield should never have been marketed. So did Connie Deemer's physician. She was so angered by what she had learned about the Shield since inserting it in Connie, that she testified she wouldn't put it in a dog.

The testimony that Post believed swayed the jury most, however, came from a biostatistician whom Post brought in to discuss the statistics revealed in Clark's June 1970 memo—the "secret" memo. The biostatistician stated that the true pregnancy rate of the Shield, using Davis' own life table calculations, was actually five percent. In other words, the pregnancy rate claims that A. H. Robins had been making in its promotional materials for the Shield were 500 percent off the mark. A woman was five times more likely to become pregnant with the Shield than the claims indicated. Instead of one woman out of 100 getting pregnant wearing the Shield, the true figure was five women out of 100.

The A. H. Robins argument that Connie's pregnancy was not its fault because the company had never guaranteed that the Shield would work 100 percent of the time was successfully refuted by the biostatistician's testimony. Connie had known there was a risk she might become pregnant while using the Shield, but she had not been told the true risk. If she had been told the Shield carried a 5 percent risk of pregnancy, she might have chosen some other form of birth control. Even the diaphragm has a better pregnancy rate.

For its defense, A. H. Robins brought in nine expert witnesses, including eight medical doctors and one engineer. But the testimony they presented was sometimes conflicting. Fred Clark, for example, testified in a deposition before the trial that the memo he had written after visiting with Hugh Davis in Baltimore was accurate. But at the trial, he changed his testimony and said that his memo was full of errors. In fact, he said his first error had been scribbling out the memo at all.

While Siefkin was arguing A. H. Robins' case in court, Tuttle was desperately working behind the scenes trying to convince one of his key witnesses, Hugh Davis, to tell the truth.

When the first Shield-related lawsuits had come in at A. H. Robins, Tuttle had turned to the medical department and asked for support, and as part of that request asked for "the one guy that knows more about this than anybody else, and that's Hugh Davis." The two men were put in touch and Tuttle began writing letters and talking to Davis about the Shield. But it was more than a year later, in the fall of 1974, that Tuttle began to realize that Davis and A. H. Robins weren't telling him everything he needed to know about the Shield.

Tuttle was defending the Shield in the California case that had ended in a mistrial when he realized that the facts weren't fitting together as he thought they should. In the opening phases of the California trial the lawyer for the woman suing A. H. Robins "appeared to have knowledge that was inconsistent with what I thought I knew about the whole history of the problem," Tuttle said. The woman's lawyer kept insisting that Davis had an ownership interest in the Shield.

A. H. Robins officials had told Tuttle only that Davis was a paid consultant and "that was the leverage that I had to insist that he cooperate with me in educating me and appearing as an expert witness." Indeed, Davis was paid more than $1,800 for his work in the Tuttle case.

As the California trial progressed, Tuttle became increasingly concerned that Davis wasn't telling the truth about his financial interest in the Shield. Finally, in October 1974, Tuttle told the attorneys he was working with in the trial that he was going to call Robert Cohn, one of the original partners in the Dalkon Corporation, and "lean on him" to find out what Davis' true business relationship with A. H. Robins and the Shield was. Tuttle has testified that Cohn was reluctant to detail how royalties from the Shield were being divided among the original Dalkon partners, but that Cohn did confirm that Davis was receiving royalties from the Shield. Cohn, however, has denied ever having such a conversation with Tuttle, although he does recall acrimonious phone calls with Tuttle about other Shield matters.

The news that Davis had a financial interest in the Shield was more than an embarrassment for Tuttle. His key witness, he now knew, had lied under oath in depositions and at Senator Gaylord Nelson's Pill hearings. (Davis later said that he had lied under orders from Tuttle—a claim Tuttle denies.)

One of those depositions was taken on February 20, 1974, by Bradley Post in Richmond in preparation for the Deemer case. Post questioned Davis directly about his financial interest in the Shield:

POST: "Do you have any agreement with Mr. Lerner of the Dalkon Corporation whereby you receive any of the royalties he receives from the Robins Company's sales of the Dalkon Shield?"

DAVIS: "I do not."

POST: "Have you ever?"

DAVIS: "No."

POST: "Have you ever owned any stock in the Dalkon Corporation?"

DAVIS: "I do not own any stock in the Dalkon Corporation."

Post wasn't going to let him slide off the question that easily. "I said have you *ever* owned any stock in the Dalkon Corporation," he repeated.

Davis paused. "I was trying to recall the events around 1968," he said. "Mr. Lerner offered me some stock in this corporation, and my decision at that time was not to hold it, because I felt there would be a conflict of interest. I did not feel—"

Post interrupted him. "Why did you feel there would be a conflict of interest?"

"Because I did not feel I should be in a position of testing and evaluating a device in which on one side I was functioning as an evaluator and on the other side I was in a capacity to, as a private individual, profit from participating in the corporation," was Davis' answer.

Of course, that is exactly what Davis had done.

Later, Post returned to the question of who was financially benefitting from the Shield.

"Do you know whether Robins Company pays any royalty to anyone for the Dalkon Shield which they purchased from the Dalkon Corporation?" he asked Davis.

"I believe from conversations with Mr. Lerner that he is receiving some form of payment from the Robins Company to which he sold his interest," answered Davis.

Davis forgot to add that he, too, was receiving payments from A. H. Robins. At the time of that deposition, he had received more than $300,000 in royalties from the Dalkon Shield.

Tuttle chose not to confront Davis immediately about this earlier deposition, but said he did tell his boss back at A. H. Robins, William Forrest (the company's vice-president and general counsel), about his problem with Davis' testimony. Tuttle said Forrest's response to the revelation was, "Deal with it."

After the California case ended in a mistrial, Tuttle confronted Davis about his interest in the Shield. The two were on an airplane flying to Wichita for the Deemer trial. Tuttle later recounted the discussion: "Basically, I told [Davis] that he'd cut me adrift once and I didn't want it to happen again, and that irrespective of how embarrassing it may be, that he had to testify honestly and accurately." Davis reacted "in an uncomplimentary fashion," Tuttle said, "and I let him vent it and then told him that . . . he either do as I was requesting or that there would be some unfortunate results."

While on the stand during Connie Deemer's trial, Davis revealed for the first time—albeit somewhat vaguely—his financial interest in the Shield.

But Davis continued to be difficult to deal with, Tuttle said. "Davis had an explanation for everything. He could explain why black was white and conversely. It didn't satisfy me, but it had to be dealt with."

Testifying a decade after the Deemer case about his relationship with Davis, Tuttle said, "Well, looking back, Davis was on so many sides of every issue that I have great difficulty now separating out truth from fiction in all that he told me over a period of years."

The jury in Connie Deemer's case apparently had no trouble separating out the truth. On February 8, 1975, it awarded Connie $10,000 in compensatory damages and $75,000 in punitive damages from A. H. Robins. It also found Connie's doctor not liable for damages.

At the conclusion of the trial, attorney Robert Siefkin wrote a letter to

Aetna Casualty and Surety Company, A. H. Robins' insurance company, strongly condemning A. H. Robins' acquisition of the Shield and Tuttle's handling of Connie Deemer's case.

"The evidence, as I see it," Siefkin wrote to Aetna officials, "shows they [Robins officials] bought a contraceptive device without adequate investigation and then they did little or no testing on the device and sold the hell out of it." That was a strong statement from an attorney who had just spent months defending A. H. Robins.

"It was a long letter," Tuttle later recalled, "and Mr. Siefkin expressed himself in strong language, blasted me as I recall. Not only targeting me, but other folks from Robins, and in effect justifying to the Aetna, not to Robins, but to the Aetna, why the case had gone sour." Tuttle has said he believes the derogatory letter had been written because, "in many instances when an important case is lost, every monkey heads for his own tree, and there was considerable finger-pointing in respect [to] whose fault it was."

Several weeks after the jury ruled in favor of Connie Deemer, Tuttle and other A. H. Robins officials flew to Hartford, Connecticut, to discuss the implications of the verdict with Aetna representatives.

Tuttle has said he was later told by his boss, William Forrest, that Aetna officials "had demanded my scalp for losing the Deemer case." Tuttle has also said he was subsequently fired by Forrest, but managed to keep his job when A. H. Robins' president William Zimmer intervened on his behalf. Forrest and Zimmer say Tuttle was never fired, but was relieved of handling Dalkon Shield cases.

Tuttle left the company about a year after the jury ruled in favor of Connie Deemer. He took with him a secret he would not reveal for nine years.

Claims and Counterclaims

"The Dalkon Shield is not a dead issue, at least not to the 600,000 women who it is estimated are still wearing them."
—Attorney Aaron Levine, speaking before the FDA's Obstetrical and Gynecological Device Classification Panel, December 1977.

By mid-1975 the troubling first chapters of the Dalkon Shield story had been completed. The IUD was permanently off the market, new device legislation was gaining momentum in Congress, and A. H. Robins realized it faced many years of tough and expensive legal battles.

Across the country, lawyers were awakening to the potential of the products liability cases that the Shield had created. With women wearing the device numbering in the hundreds of thousands, many attorneys saw the Shield as a financial bonanza.

A. H. Robins, too, realized it was facing years of legal problems far beyond anything its small, in-house staff of lawyers could handle. The company had already paid more than $1.5 million for the settlement of lawsuits, legal fees, and other expenses because of the Shield. So, in mid-1975 the company hired Richmond's largest and most prestigious law firm, McGuire, Woods and Battle. It was the law firm where then–A. H. Robins President William Zimmer had worked before joining the pharmaceutical company. That Zimmer turned to his old law firm for help signaled the seriousness with which he viewed the coming chapter of the Dalkon Shield story.

In Rockville, Maryland, 100 miles north of Richmond, FDA officials continued their efforts to try to determine just how much of a danger IUDs really posed. The Shield was off the market for good, but no clear-cut, convincing scientific data on the safety of the Shield or other IUDs had yet been collected. The agency was also busy trying to complete its classification program for thousands of medical devices. And the ongoing effort to get new, stronger device legislation through Congress had yet to succeed.

But while A. H. Robins was preparing for the onslaught of lawsuits, and while the FDA was trying to resolve the growing debate about IUD safety, hundreds of thousands of women continued to wear the Dalkon Shield.

The device was, as a judge would later say, "a deadly depth charge in their wombs, ready to explode at any time."

Before Connie Deemer's case, most lawsuits involving the Dalkon Shield were, in the words of A. H. Robins' own attorney, Roger Tuttle, "relatively unsophisticated products-liability suits grounded on the theory of uterine perforation."

Plaintiffs' attorneys, representing women who believed they had been harmed by the Shield, argued that the device had a faulty design that had allowed it to push its way through the uterus into the abdominal cavity. They claimed the women were entitled to collect damages for the perforation itself (which usually necessitated surgical repair) and for the "unwanted" pregnancy that occurred because the device was in the abdomen rather than in the uterus, protecting against pregnancy.

Pelvic inflammatory disease (PID) was also the basis of many of the early lawsuits. Howard Tatum had not yet completed and made public his study that first showed that the Shield's tail string was multifilament and thus a potential wick for bacteria. So plaintiffs' attorneys in these early PID cases could only argue that the device had irritated the lining of the uterus and, as a result, had aggravated a minor existing disease or inflammation.

A. H. Robins defended both perforation and PID lawsuits by blaming the women's doctors. In perforation cases, the company argued, as it had done in Connie Deemer's trial, the injury had occurred because the doctor had hurried during insertion, shoving the IUD through the uterus. A. H. Robins did not acknowledge, however, that the Shield's design and rigid inserter stick may have contributed to these perforations, nor that some of its employees had expressed concern about the device's propensity for perforations within months of its marketing.

As for claims involving PID, A. H. Robins argued that doctors had not thoroughly examined their patients for a pre-existing infection. Any negligence was the fault of the doctors, said the company, not of A. H. Robins. In fact, if a woman didn't sue her doctor in addition to A. H. Robins, the company would file its own cross-claim against the doctor. As it turned out, this wasn't a good idea.

"In retrospect this was poor tactical judgment because it drove Robins's natural ally, the prescribing physician, to cooperate with the plantiff [sic] and oppose Robins," Tuttle later wrote in a law journal. "The net result was that invariably the physician denied receiving the promotional literature and instructions and blamed Robins for leading him astray in treating his patient."

Although A. H. Robins risked alienating doctors with this tactic, the overall legal strategy worked fairly well during the first years of Dalkon Shield litigation. Damages were, for the most part, kept under $10,000 for each claim settled before 1975. None of these cases actually went to trial. "Statistically, by injury, well over 50 per cent of the cases were perforation," recalled Tuttle, "35 per cent were unwanted children, and the balance was a mélange of theories, including one exotic dancer who claimed a cesarian section for delivery of a live birth was caused by the device and the resultant scars left her disfigured and lowered her economic value as an exotic dancer."

Then Connie Deemer's suit came along, and with it the discovery of Fred Clark's "secret memo." After the memo was revealed, Tuttle said, plaintiffs' lawyers began arguing to judges and juries that "Robins could not be trusted, that it was covering up, and that it had misled physicians and consumers and the FDA."

The ongoing negative publicity about the Shield, especially the 1974 Centers for Disease Control study that revealed a close association between septic abortions and the Shield, led to what Tuttle described as a "geometric progression" of lawsuits. By April 1976, less than a year after A. H. Robins had abandoned all plans to market the Shield again, 533 suits demanding $480 million in punitive and compensatory damages were pending before courts throughout the country.

As more and more suits were filed, more and more attorneys became interested in the litigation. Soon lawyers for the women were forming competing groups, with each faction trying to become the national lead group for women claiming damages from the Shield.

The group that finally won control was headed by Bradley Post. He obtained an order from the Judicial Panel on Multi-District Litigation (MDL) that transferred for pretrial purposes all the federal cases to the U.S. District Court for the District of Kansas, Wichita Division. This meant that all attorneys who filed Dalkon Shield cases in federal courts throughout the country would now go through Post to obtain the materials and expertise they needed to try the cases. And Post would be responsible for gathering those materials—taking depositions, wading through the thousands of documents in Richmond, and so on. He became the national clearinghouse for Dalkon Shield litigation. In return, Post would receive a fee—reportedly $400—from each case filed in federal court and processed through him.

Such an arrangement is not unusual in mass litigation, because it saves everyone involved time and money. In the Dalkon Shield cases it saved attorneys representing the women the incredibly tedious and expensive task of duplicating the efforts of attorneys who had gone before them. And it saved A. H. Robins the considerable nuisance of having hordes of attorneys knocking on their door asking for documents and depositions that had already been produced elsewhere.

The Dalkon Shield MDL discovery process in 1976 was supervised by U.S. Judge Frank Theis of Kansas. Under him, Post put together massive files of documents. He also took depositions of A. H. Robins officials, which, when completed and transcribed, numbered into thousands of pages.

When the first MDL discovery process was completed in 1976, A. H. Robins said it had handed over all the documents it believed plaintiffs' attorneys were entitled to. Most of the judges and lawyers involved took them at their word. It would be nearly a decade later before it became apparent that everything had not been handed over.

It wasn't long after Post's success with Connie Deemer's case that some lawyers saw a quick way to make a profit on the Dalkon Shield. After all, more than two million women—a huge potential market of clients—had worn the device.

Finding those women, however, was another matter. In the first few years of Shield litigation, lawyers basically had to wait for women to find them. Then, in 1977, the United States Supreme Court ruled that attorneys could advertise routine legal services.

Two of the attorneys who first took advantage of that ruling in connection with Dalkon Shield litigation were Robert Appert and Gerald Pyle. By the end of 1977, these two Minnesota attorneys had distributed more than 500 copies of a brochure that announced: "Women who have used Dalkon Shield may be entitled to Financial Compensation." They also mailed a circular to friends, clients, and former clients, inviting women to call their law firm if they had ever experienced problems with the Shield.

In addition, Pyle encouraged a college student to undertake a research project on the device. Advertisements were placed in two small community papers, offering $10 to any woman who had worn the Dalkon Shield and who was willing to talk about her experience with it. After interviewing the women, the student referred them to Pyle's law firm. One woman who didn't follow up on the referral said Pyle later called her several times.

These advertising schemes worked well. By the end of 1978, Appert and Pyle had about 550 Dalkon Shield cases, for an incredible 16 percent of the total number filed in the United States. Shield cases now made up one-half of the firm's caseload.

Appert and Pyle were not especially aggressive litigating attorneys, however. Other plaintiffs' attorneys criticized them for filing claims with A. H. Robins' insurer, the Aetna Casualty and Surety Company, instead of filing lawsuits against the company in court, and for settling the claims quickly without even threatening to take A. H. Robins to court. The firm took no depositions, nor did it attempt to collect any documents from A. H. Robins.

During 1978, Appert and Pyle's settlements for their Dalkon Shield clients averaged $10,000—a full $10,000 less than the settlements attorneys elsewhere in the country were averaging by then.

One woman revealed to a *Minneapolis Tribune* reporter that Pyle had tried to pressure her into accepting an offer of $3,800 from A. H. Robins' insurer, the Aetna Casualty and Surety Company. "You're not being realistic," she said Pyle told her after she rejected the offer and indicated she wanted to take her case to court. "You should jump at the chance before they get mad and change their minds. You don't have a case. They don't have to give you a dime. You're lucky you're getting anything." Pyle then told her, she said, that he would drop her as his client if she didn't accept Aetna's offer. The woman found another attorney several weeks later who got her another offer from Aetna—this time for $10,000, which the woman finally accepted.

But it was their advertising tactics, not their unaggressive handling of Dalkon Shield cases, that got Appert and Pyle in trouble with their legal peers. Minnesota's Lawyers Professional Responsibility Board questioned the ethics of the ads and took the matter to the state's court. But in December 1981, the Minnesota Supreme Court ruled that Appert and Pyle had not violated ethical rules for attorney advertising in their solicitation of Dalkon Shield clients.

By that time, however, the two attorneys were out of the Dalkon Shield picture. A. H. Robins had seen to that. The company had earlier filed a motion to have Appert and Pyle disqualified from Dalkon Shield cases because the two lawyers had allegedly had an adjuster from Aetna on their payroll. As A. H. Robins' insurance company, Aetna covered A. H. Robins' losses in Dalkon Shield cases. For attorneys who were filing scores of claims against A. H. Robins to have an Aetna employee on their payroll created, at the very least, serious conflict of interest problems.

At the same time another Minnesota attorney, Norman Perl, was being charged with striking behind-the-scenes deals with the same Aetna insurance adjuster to settle women's Dalkon Shield claims for a set amount. It was alleged that Perl split the fee with the adjuster in "a system of payoffs and kickbacks."

Perl was later acquitted of these charges, but was ordered to return $350,000 in legal fees to 74 of his former Dalkon Shield clients. The court ruled he was not entitled to these fees because he did not disclose to the women his business relationship with the Aetna adjuster.

Many observers believe that A. H. Robins' attempt to get Appert and Pyle disqualified from Dalkon Shield cases was really an attempt to send a message to other attorneys who might be contemplating similar advertising schemes. The last thing in the world A. H. Robins wanted was for lawyers to alert women to the fact that they might have a case for a lawsuit against the company. Appert and Pyle fought the disqualification motion for almost a year, but finally in October 1981, they agreed to withdraw from the 400 Dalkon Shield cases they then had pending in court, claiming they could no longer afford to fight A. H. Robins on the issue.

Although Appert and Pyle can be credited with alerting many women to their legal rights concerning the Dalkon Shield, their eagerness—and the eagerness of many other attorneys across the country—to arrange low settlements that required little legal work certainly raises the question of whose best interests were being served by those settlements: the lawyers' or the women's. Indeed, in 1985 both Appert and Pyle were suspended from practicing law by the Minnesota Supreme Court after a disciplinary panel found that they had engaged in incidents of unprofessional conduct while handling Shield cases.

But not all attorneys saw the Dalkon Shield merely as a way of making money. Some, as they became more and more involved in the cases, were genuinely outraged by what had happened to the women. For these attorneys, their Dalkon Shield cases soon became a cause.

On the morning of December 5, 1977, Washington, D.C., attorney Aaron Levine contacted FDA official Lillian Yin and said he and Wichita attorney Bradley Post wanted to make a presentation that afternoon to the agency's Obstetrical and Gynecological Device Classification Panel. Levine and Post weren't on the agenda for the meeting, but Yin, director of the FDA's division of Ob-Gyn Medical Devices and head of the Ob-Gyn Device Classification Panel, quickly scheduled them in. She gave them 10 minutes.

Levine was an abrasive, no-nonsense attorney. In 1976 he had, at consumer activist Ralph Nader's recommendation, been appointed to serve as a consumer representative on the FDA's Anesthesia Device Committee, one of a number of device committees the FDA had set up to classify the thousands of medical devices on the market. In his private law practice, Levine represented women who were suing A. H. Robins because of the Dalkon Shield.

Both Levine and Post believed that even though the Dalkon Shield was off the market, it remained dangerous to the estimated 600,000 women who were still wearing it.

Since October 1974, several months after A. H. Robins had suspended marketing of the Shield, the FDA had taken the position that, until better scientific information could be developed, it was all right for doctors to leave the Dalkon Shield in women who were not having any problems with it. This position had been recommended by a special Ad Hoc Committee of physicians that had studied the medical literature on IUDs for the FDA.

Levine and Post, however, wanted the FDA to quit waiting for more studies and immediately tell women wearing the Shield to have it removed.

"The Dalkon Shield is not a dead issue, at least to the 600,000 women who it is estimated are still wearing them," Levine told the five members of the panel. He then introduced Post, describing him as "the most knowledgeable man on the Dalkon Shield outside the Robins organization." Post, knowing he was limited to 10 minutes, quickly told the panel why he was there—to urge the FDA to immediately tell women to remove the Dalkon Shield.

"As Mr. Levine told you, the Dalkon Shield is sometimes referred to by gynecologists and obstetricians and possibly members of this organization as a dead issue," Post said, "but certainly it is not to those women still wearing it." Post told the panel that he had called upon A. H. Robins officials to issue a letter to doctors to "set the record straight concerning the modified, untested device that was promoted to the medical profession and the public beginning in January 1971."

Post was referring to a letter he had written on February 16, 1977, to Alexander Slaughter, a Richmond attorney representing A. H. Robins in Shield cases. In his letter Post pleaded with A. H. Robins to issue its own letter telling doctors to remove the Shield from women still wearing it. "It is my personal opinion and conclusion that the Dalkon shield is an inferior, dangerous and defective IUD," Post told Slaughter in the letter. "Aside from the question of whether or not my appraisal is accurate, it seems to me that Robins does have a continuing duty to withdraw previous advertising and promotional claims and to provide accurate information to the medical profession concerning efficacy of the product it marketed." A. H. Robins promotional material and advertising were based on studies of the original Shield design, not the "modified" Shield that was marketed by A. H. Robins, Post said.

Post enclosed an independent analysis of A. H. Robins' own Ten Investigator Prospective Study data on the Shield. "Any reasonable review of these studies leads to the inescapable conclusion that the pregnancy rate for the modified device promoted by Robins exceeds 5% at 12 months." Post asked A. H. Robins to issue a "Dear Doctor" letter to inform physicians that the Shield had been modified before marketing and that the "original claims were based on an earlier version" of the device. He also asked A. H. Robins to reveal the "financial interest of [Hugh] Davis and questionable nature of [the] original studies relied upon." He also asked A. H. Robins to "recommend immediate removal of devices in use."

"I consider each day until this action is taken to be a continuous, voluntary and conscious decision to withhold vital information from the medical profession and the public," Post wrote in his letter.

He had asked A. H. Robins to issue the letter, Post told the FDA panel, but the company had "not seen fit to do so." "It's my recommendation to this organization that you make a strong recommendation to Robins to send out such a letter or, in the alternative, that you put out a bulletin through the FDA that gives the true information concerning the Dalkon Shield."

Post then began a terse presentation of his case against the Shield. It was a "misbranded" device that was sold with "false and misleading advertising," he said, referring to the 1.1 percent pregnancy rate A. H. Robins used to promote the Shield. The actual pregnancy rate was about five percent, Post said.

Post also raised the problem of the Shield's wicking tail string. "A. H.

Robins received its first notice of possible wicking problems 12 days after purchasing the device," Post said. "They chose not to do anything about the tail string of the device because the orders exceeded demand and production schedules were critical to them." A. H. Robins, he said, had studied Shield tail strings from devices taken from women in San Francisco and Houston. "They tested these devices and they found in each instance that there were viable bacteria within the sheath of those devices removed from women."

"These matters have never been made public," Post said. "They haven't been brought to the attention of the FDA." He told the panel that in April 1975, Fred Clark, Robins' medical director, had appeared before the FDA Ad Hoc Committee and had been asked if private studies had been done with the Shield. "And the answer was given that there had not, and this came up in connection with migration perforation and also infection," Post said. "Now the fact is that Robins began, eight months after national marketing, a two-year baboon safety study. It was completed. It yielded about a 30 percent perforation migration rate and a kill rate of one animal in eight from either the perforation or infection. That information was available at the time of that April 1975 open hearing when those questions were asked, but it was not brought to the attention of the [Ad Hoc Committee]."

Post moved quickly to his recommendations, which were similar to those he'd proposed to A. H. Robins months earlier. First, anyone wearing the Dalkon Shield should have it removed. If a woman wants to keep her Shield, she should use contraceptive foam for part of her cycle (to avoid the dangers of becoming pregnant with the Shield in place). The medical profession should be told the original claims for the Shield are false, he said, and doctors should know that the man who did the study upon which the efficacy claims are based, Hugh Davis, "owned 35 percent of the device from day one." Doctors should also be told that the device that was sold was substantially different from the device Davis tested. Finally, A. H. Robins should be required to withdraw the statements it made, when it stopped marketing the Shield, claiming the device was safe and effective.

Milton Heller, the consumer liaison to the panel, wanted to talk to Post about his statement but was quickly cut off by Yin. "May I now ask why this can't be discussed?" Heller said after Post completed his statement.

"If they [Post and Levine] had wanted us to discuss it they should have let us know way ahead and we will allot time for and send the material out ahead of time," Yin explained. "Because we do have other material that if it is going to be discussed the panel should have all the material ahead of time."

Heller wanted to talk to Post. "These are fairly serious charges," he said. "Do you intend to definitely schedule it for the next meeting?"

"No," Yin replied. "First of all, I really think this should be brought to the FDA first [instead of to the panel], and then . . . [the] FDA would have to make up their mind which way it is going to handle the situation." Besides, Yin said, it wouldn't be fair to the panel members—especially the new ones—to "jump into this" without more background material.

Thomas Trussell, Jr., a consultant to the panel, spoke up in support of Heller. "Why couldn't it be done at our next meeting?" he asked.

"First of all," Yin said, "the FDA would have to decide what type of meeting we are going to have, either another open hearing or the ad hoc committee, because it was not discussed; just the device committee. We invited the drug panel of the ad hoc committee."

Post's statement on the Shield was beginning to disappear into a bureaucratic quagmire. Heller tried again. "But the background material can be disseminated before the next meeting."

"Yes," Yin said. "if FDA does decide that that is the right thing to do for one panel meeting."

Heller persisted. "We could put this on the agenda. I might wonder if Mr. Post can return with some other scientists if possible?" Post volunteered to bring back several scientists to back up his criticism of the Shield.

Richard Dickey, a panel member who had been very critical of the FDA's handling of the Dalkon Shield issue when the device was first taken off the market, said Post was providing "new information" that should be looked into after it had been "introduced through the channels of FDA." Post began to discuss why the FDA had not moved against the Shield as it had with the Majzlin Spring, but the discussion was abruptly ended.

"I think the Chair takes the prerogative of discontinuing this conversation, all of which is interesting and pertinent except that we have a tremendous amount of work we have to do this afternoon," said Dr. Charlotte Kerr, who headed the panel. "And therefore we move on to the next subject."

The next day Fred Clark had a memo from Fletcher Owen on his desk at A. H. Robins. George Smith, a member of the Pharmaceutical Manufacturers Association, had heard about the Post-Levine statement and had called Owen to tell him about it. Smith had gotten the information second-hand, and somewhere in the retelling, Bradley Post was left out of the story. The memo outlined the charges that Post had made, but attributed them to Levine. Owen told Clark about Levine's request that the FDA issue a letter to doctors urging removal of the Shield. "Dr. Dickey, a panel member, appeared to be the strongest supporter of Mr. Levine's proposal," Owen told Clark. "It was suggested that the matter might be considered at the next scheduled meeting in April, 1978."

Owen suggested that A. H. Robins contact Yin and ask for a transcript of the entire meeting, and if the transcript wasn't immediately available, "we should ask to hear any prepared tapes of the session."

Post and Levine had succeeded in creating a minor stir at A. H. Robins headquarters with their presentation, but they accomplished little else. The FDA never did send out the letter they asked for.

Yin later explained the FDA inaction on the Post-Levine statement by saying there was "no scientific data" presented. "We had a long dissertation on what's what," she said, "by two attorneys who were suing Robins. We can't judge based on that. We had a CDC [Centers for Disease Control] study saying it [the Shield] could be left in. Do you think we can use a lawyer's statement and [go to Robins and doctors with a removal letter] and say here it is. You cannot say there is a lawsuit against something so you'd better remove that product."

There were clearly strong concerns within the FDA about the Shield, Yin said. After all, she pointed out, it was the FDA that asked A. H. Robins to remove the device from the market in 1974 after learning about the relationship between the Shield and septic abortions. But FDA guidelines for allowing the Shield back on the market had been issued in 1974 to deal with that problem, she said, and the best information the agency had when Post and Levine appeared indicated the Shield had a PID rate of about five percent, which wasn't too high by agency standards.

"The FDA would be the laughing stock" if it had "run around like a chicken with its head cut off" trying to get the Shield removed from women without the scientific data to back it up, she said. "I don't want sympathy," Yin said, "but do you know how difficult it is being the FDA? We tend to be conservative and we're always getting yelled and screamed at. You have to have the science."

Years later, Levine was still furious with Yin for not telling physicians to remove the Shield from women in 1977. "She is responsible for hysterectomies in 5,000 women," Levine said in 1984. "You can tell her I said that."

For the next several years the FDA continued to sponsor studies on IUDs, particularly in relation to PID. Based on information coming in to the agency from its advisory committees and medical studies, the FDA finally decided to issue warnings about IUDs—first in a 1978 Drug Bulletin and then in a 1979 Consumer Memo. In both instances the FDA informed physicians and the public that "PID is three to five times more likely to occur in users of IUDs than nonusers; and IUD contraception carries a risk of PID which may lead to infertility."

In December 1978, the FDA released its update of its 1968 IUD report and its conclusions essentially echoed what the agency had been telling the public: IUDs have risks, but generally are an acceptable form of contraception. In February 1980, the medical device classification process that had begun in 1971 finally was completed. The new medical device regulations, strengthened by Congress in 1976, said that even IUDs that were classified as devices had to undergo pre-market approval by the agency. It was just such pre-market approval that the Shield had escaped when it had been classified as a device rather than a drug in 1972.

Fletcher Owen arrived at Lillian Yin's office in one of the several FDA buildings scattered around the Washington suburb of Rockville, Maryland, on September 24, 1980. He carried with him a letter that A. H. Robins would mail out to 200,000 physicians the next day—a letter that quickly became known as "Dear Doctor Number 2." Owen gave a copy of the letter to Yin.

"Dear Doctor," the letter began, "Domestic distribution of the Dalkon Shield by the A. H. Robins Company was discontinued in June, 1974. Subsequently, we have concurred with the majority of medical opinion relative to IUDs in suggesting that women who continue to use the Dalkon Shield without problems or difficulties need not have it removed."

The letter continued on for several more paragraphs, describing new research on PID in women who were "long-term" IUD wearers. One type of PID seemed to be particularly related to long-term use of an IUD, the letter noted. This infection was caused by a bacteria known as Actinomyces israelii, and "is usually insidious in onset and clinical symptoms may be absent until a pelvic mass is noted on examination. By this time, advanced disease of the tubes, ovaries or uterus may be present [meaning a woman could be sterile].

"The infection has been reported in users of a variety of IUD types. Recent reports have indicated that the problem can be minimized by replacing inert IUDs [those that don't contain substances that react with the body, such as copper] at periodic intervals, generally not exceeding three years."

Finally, in the last paragraph, the letter got to its main point: "Since any present users of the Dalkon Shield are in the long-term use category, we now recommend removal of this IUD from any of your patients who continue to use it, even though they may not be experiencing any pelvic symptoms at this time. We further suggest that the removed IUD and adherent material be submitted to a clinical pathology laboratory for examination for organisms consistent with [PID]."

The letter was calling for essentially what Bradley Post and Aaron Levine had asked for three years earlier—removing the Shield from women.

Yin didn't like the A. H. Robins letter. She told Owen that the FDA was planning amendments to IUD labeling requirements that would alert doctors to the very infection the A. H. Robins letter warned about. She told him the FDA would not endorse the "Dear Doctor" letter and would begin a review of A. H. Robins' recommendation that Dalkon Shields be removed from women to "determine its validity."

Yin also told Owen that the letter could be interpreted as a recall of the Shield by A. H. Robins. That could have serious legal implications for A. H. Robins, because in hundreds of lawsuits, the company was arguing that there was nothing wrong with the Shield. That would be a difficult argument to make if the FDA ruled that the company had recalled the product.

Owen told Yin that it wasn't a recall, but that A. H. Robins was acting as a responsible pharmaceutical company by calling doctors' and the public's attention to new developments reported in medical literature. The next day A. H. Robins began mailing out 200,000 copies of the letter to doctors, medical schools, and state health departments.

After years of steadfastly maintaining the Shield was a safe and effective product, why was A. H. Robins suddenly urging doctors to remove it? Paul Teitell and Robert Turk, both FDA investigators stationed in Richmond, visited with A. H. Robins officials and looked through company records to get a full explanation for the letter. In a memo to the FDA in December 1980, they detailed what they had been told by A. H. Robins officials: Robins had first become concerned about the special PID problem at a medical conference in New Orleans in February 1980. At the conference Dr. Waldemar Schmidt of the University of Texas Medical School in Houston reported on a study he was conducting on the relationship between the length of time an IUD had been in a woman's body and the increased risk of PID.

A. H. Robins' medical department contacted Schmidt and other "undisclosed" medical authorities, the FDA inspectors said, and received an abstract of the study about to be published by Schmidt.

In July 1980, E. Claiborne Robins, Jr., was told of the new problems with long-term wearing of an IUD, and he asked for a more thorough investigation, the FDA inspectors were told.

In August 1980, after receiving the completed Schmidt study, Owen flew to Houston to "verify Dr. Schmidt's findings." That visit was apparently enough to convince Owen that the Shield should be removed from women. The FDA inspectors were told by the company that work on the "Dear Doctor Number 2" letter was begun in late August and finally printed on September 18 and 19, then forwarded to a mailing service on the 22 to be mailed on the 25.

It was after work on the letter had begun, the inspectors were told, that Owen became aware of a second study that indicated the same problem that Dr. Schmidt had noted. The study was published in the August 1980 issue of the *British Medical Journal* and Owen decided to cite it in the "Dear Doctor Number 2" letter.

But the FDA remained suspicious of the letter. First, the letter implicated all IUDs, not just the Dalkon Shield. The letter said the PID infection had been reported "in users of a variety of IUD types," and added that "recent reports have indicated that the problem can be minimized by replacing inert IUDs at periodic intervals."

That, the FDA said, could be read as suggesting that all IUDs, not just the Shield, should be removed from women. The FDA's official position was that doctors didn't have to remove even the Shield from women, much less other "inert" IUDs. (It had a different position on IUDs that were classified as drugs; they interact with the body and were supposed to be replaced every three years, according to the FDA.) If the information stated in A. H. Robins' letter were true, Yin said later, then the FDA "should have dragged everybody in and removed all IUDs."

The FDA suspected other reasons for the letter. There were rumors that the CBS program "60 Minutes" was about to air an exposé about the Shield, and the FDA wondered if the "Dear Doctor Number 2" letter might have been sent to head off the anticipated bad publicity. A. H. Robins told FDA Inspector Teitell the letter had "nothing to do with the anticipated" broadcast. (On April 19, 1981, "60 Minutes" did air a segment highly critical of the Shield.)

In April 1981, an FDA official suggested yet another motive. In an April 22 memo, Dr. Yvonne Wilson, the medical officer for the FDA's division of Ob-Gyn and Radiology Devices, told Yin that the agency's Bureau of Medical Devices "suspects that A. H. Robins' actions may be due to an attempt to reduce its liability in the multitude of suits which they continue to be involved in by using this still controversial issue to effect a removal of their product without calling for a recall."

The FDA, Yin said, decided to keep silent. If A. H. Robins wanted to get the Shield out of women, for whatever reason, then the FDA wouldn't object, she said.

It was not until 1983, two years later, that Yin began to realize that A. H. Robins officials had not been telling her all they knew about the dangers of the Shield.

She had worked closely with Owen and other A. H. Robins officials over the years, she said, yet it wasn't until documents supporting a petition against the Shield were filed with the FDA in April 1983 by the Women's Health Network that Yin realized A. H. Robins had not told her what they knew about the Shield's wicking problems.

What was so "objectionable" to her, Yin said, was that the company "knew about the problem with wicking from day one and didn't tell us. I was angry when I found out about it. In 1974 they acted so innocent."

17

The Minnesota Experience

"I said regardless of how bright [the Robins attorneys] are, they have to know that we are totally committed to the cause and that we'll leave no stone unturned. We're coming after them and we're not going to relent. All fronts. We're going to broaden the attack, going to go after their directors and officers and put the same questions to them that they put to the women. Going to go after Aetna, go after their outside directors, their law firms and let them know they're in a war and they can never, ever doubt it."
— Michael Ciresi, plaintiffs' attorney.

The winter of 1984 was a bone-chiller for Minnesota, the kind of winter even natives grumble about. For 35 days, temperatures dipped below zero degrees, and the state had one of its heaviest snowfalls of the century.

Yet despite the bitter cold and heavy snow, Minnesota became a hotbed for Dalkon Shield litigation that winter, with lawyers flying frequently and frantically between Richmond and Minneapolis, gathering documents, taking depositions, fighting heated legal skirmishes in and out of the courtroom.

By spring, when most of the legal heat had dissipated, the A. H. Robins' icy wall of defense, a wall that had been carefully constructed during more than 10 years of litigation, began to show cracks. Deep cracks.

The source of those cracks could be traced back to the fall of 1982, when Minnesota found its courts threatened with hundreds of Dalkon Shield lawsuits—more, in fact, than any other single state.

This large number of lawsuits was due in large part to the advertising efforts of Robert Appert and Gerald Pyle, the two Minnesota attorneys who had been brought before the Minnesota Supreme Court for violating professional ethics. Although Appert and Pyle withdrew from Dalkon Shield litigation in 1981, their 500 or so remaining cases had been turned over, under court supervision, to another Minnesota law firm. That firm quickly filed the cases in court, along with about 100 cases referred to it by other attorneys.

The law firm that took on those cases was Robins, Zelle, Larson, and Kaplan. The third largest law firm in Minnesota, Robins-Zelle had a reputation for being aggressive and persistent, willing to risk large amounts of time and money to pursue multi-year litigation. Much of this aggressiveness stemmed from the youthfulness of its lawyers. Although founded in 1938, the average age of its partners at the beginning of its involvement in the Dalkon Shield litigation was 41; the average age of all its attorneys was only 34.

Robins-Zelle specialized in industrial disasters. Among the major lawsuits it had handled prior to the Dalkon Shield cases were such tragic disasters as the MGM Grand Hotel fire in Las Vegas, Nevada, in November 1980, and the collapse of a skyway in the Hyatt Regency Hotel in Kansas City, Missouri, in July 1981.

The Robins-Zelle firm had also helped pioneer the products liability field of law. In 1960, one of the firm's founders, Solly Robins, won a landmark case involving a girl who had been scalded by hot water from a defectively designed vaporizer. The case established the legal doctrine that proving negligence—failure to use reasonable care to protect others from harm—on the part of a manufacturer is unnecessary to establish liability; all that needs to be proven is that the product had a defective design.

Still, it was the Dalkon Shield cases that really brought Robins-Zelle national attention. Before 1981, Robins-Zelle had never tried an IUD case, much less one involving the Dalkon Shield. The firm had been contacted from time to time by women who claimed Dalkon Shield injuries, but it felt the cases were too involved to be handled on an individual basis. Robins-Zelle referred the cases to other Minnesota attorneys specializing in Shield cases.

Then along came the Appert and Pyle controversy. Robins-Zelle suddenly found itself being offered—and accepting—hundreds of Dalkon Shield clients. Although the firm had long been involved in mass litigation, it had never handled a class of clients this large. From a logistical standpoint alone, these Dalkon Shield cases would involve a tremendous commitment of time and resources.

But even Robins-Zelle couldn't have guessed just how massive that commitment would be. For by the time it finished its first Dalkon Shield trial, the law firm would spend more than $900,000 in out-of-pocket expenses and another $2 million in lawyers' time.

In the fall of 1982, all Dalkon Shield cases filed in Minnesota's federal court were assigned to U.S. District Judge Donald Alsop. A former defense attorney with a conservative bent, Alsop made it clear that a Dalkon Shield case was going to be tried in Minnesota—and tried soon. He didn't want the cases to create a logjam in Minnesota's federal court.

Until almost the last moment, however, no one knew which of the Dalkon Shield cases would be the first to go to trial. Robins-Zelle attorneys believe it was apparent from the start, however, that Alsop wanted it to be one of their cases. Of the first 50 cases Alsop had lined up for trial, Robins-Zelle attorney Michael Ciresi points out, almost three-fourths belonged to Robins-Zelle.

"He knew that the first case would have a significant impact on the future course of the litigation here in Minnesota," says Ciresi, one of the Robins-Zelle attorneys who eventually tried the case. "I think he wanted to make sure he wasn't sending the St. Luke's Grade School against Notre Dame."

But even Robins-Zelle's team of attorneys didn't anticipate that the game would run into overtime, that what they thought would be an eight-day trial would drag on for three months. The first hint of trouble ahead came in the fall of 1982 as Robins-Zelle attorneys began preparing for trial (still not knowing which case was going to be tried). A. H. Robins was fighting them at every turn. Pretrial discovery proved exceptionally tedious, even for a complex products liability case. Robins-Zelle attorneys had seen nothing like it before. A. H. Robins objected to almost every one of the thousands of documents Robins-Zelle wanted admitted into evidence. And it used an objection that Robins-Zelle thought was flimsy at best: The documents, argued A. H. Robins, were only "casual" memorandums that had not been produced by the employees who wrote them as part of the usual course of business. They were not, the company argued, official company documents. According to Robins-Zelle attorneys, A. H. Robins even tried to apply this objection to Fred Clark's memo of June 9, 1970, that revealed the higher pregnancy rate of Davis' study.

To answer the objections to these documents, Robins-Zelle attorneys had to find and search through trial transcripts and depositions from other Dalkon Shield cases throughout the country to locate the one reference to each document that could lay the foundation for it being admitted into court. This digging alone cost $50,000. It took the lawyers and the judge three days to resolve the first eight document disputes.

Robins-Zelle attorneys began to understand the legal strategy of A. H. Robins: Try the cases one at a time; flood the plaintiffs' attorneys with paperwork; refuse to do anything that's requested; and appeal everything. This strategy had the effect of making Dalkon Shield cases drag on and on and on—even before they reached trial. And most plaintiffs' attorneys simply did not have the resources or time for such lengthy proceedings.

By late December 1982, Robins-Zelle had picked the two attorneys it wanted to try the first case: Ciresi, 36, and Dale Larson, 45, two "local boys" who had graduated from the University of Minnesota's law school and gone on to specialize in products liability and personal injury law. Ciresi and Larson cleared away their other cases and dove into the Dalkon Shield story. Between Christmas and New Year's, they flew around the country, interviewing medical experts who might be helpful to their side and taking depositions of A. H. Robins' experts.

Ciresi's first deposition took place in New York City. He was to question Attila Toth, an assistant professor of obstetrics and gynecology at Cornell University's MacLeod Laboratory for Infertility to which A. H. Robins had paid some $98,000 to test a theory that bacteria could enter the uterus by "hitchhiking" on sperm. (Toth personally received $5,000 of that money as a salary increase.) Toth—and A. H. Robins—claimed his study had proved the theory correct.

Ciresi knew he was going to have fun with Toth and his study from the moment he met the man.

"My name is Attila Toth. In Hungary they call it 'Tot' so you can call me 'Tot' or 'Toth,' " the doctor told Ciresi.

Ciresi smiled. "My name is Ciresi," he said, "but in Italy they pronounce it 'Cherasi.' You can call me 'Ciresi' or you can call me 'Cherasi.' "

After taking Toth's deposition, Ciresi believed he could have had a field day with the professor's study in court, for not only did he think the study was "nonsensical," but that Toth had obviously slanted it from the

189

start to produce the results A. H. Robins wanted. In fact, Toth had approached A. H. Robins in 1981 about doing the study after reading news articles of Dalkon Shield lawsuits.

As one of his stated objectives for the study—written before he had begun his research and thus before he could know what the study would reveal—Toth proclaimed: "This [study] could be used to shift some of the responsibility from the IUD as a foreign body per se or the IUD string as it guides bacteria through the cervical mucus as factors that can cause pelvic inflammatory diseases. . . . We believe this study could change the legal ramifications of IUD-related litigation." So much for an unbiased study. A. H. Robins never directly presented Toth's study in any Dalkon Shield case tried by Robins-Zelle, although the company has pulled it out in other cases tried by less sophisticated attorneys.

By New Year's, both Ciresi and Larson were back in Minneapolis, trying to absorb thousands of pages of documents in preparation for the coming trial. They were amazed by what they read and frustrated by what they still did not know.

The two lawyers found the depositions taken for the MDL discovery to be deficient. Bradley Post had focused in those depositions on establishing that certain documents showed the Dalkon Shield to be defective. That was, after all, an overwhelming amount of work in itself. But Ciresi and Larson now wanted to question top officials at A. H. Robins about more than the documents.

They wanted to ask those officials, from E. Claiborne, Sr., on down, the question that had become so famous during the Watergate investigation: What did you know and when did you know it? "We were looking at the conduct of the company," explains Roger Brosnahan, a Robins-Zelle attorney who was also working on Shield cases. "That's what gets you the punitive damages."

But Ciresi and Larson weren't going to get their chance to reopen discovery, at least not at first. Judge Alsop said he wasn't going to allow new depositions to be taken of A. H. Robins officials who had already been deposed during the MDL discovery process in the mid-1970s and in early 1982. It would be too costly, he said, both in court time and in money. And, after all, the point of the MDL discovery had been to avoid just such a duplication of effort.

In January 1983, the attorneys were notified which case would be tried first. A. H. Robins had essentially chosen the case by settling all those preceding it on Judge Alsop's list.

The case was that of Brenda S., a 34-year-old waitress from Little Falls, Minnesota. On a February morning four years earlier, Brenda had doubled over with severe vaginal cramps while at work. She was rushed to a hospital where doctors performed emergency surgery, removing her right Fallopian tube, which had abscessed, and something else—the Dalkon Shield she had worn for seven years. The infection left the childless Brenda sterile.

A. H. Robins apparently thought Brenda had a weak case. They had offered her $15,000 in settlement, a figure Robins-Zelle attorneys felt was much too low for a woman who had lost her ability to have children. They believed a more appropriate settlement would be $195,000. A. H. Robins attorneys, however, believed they could convince a jury that Brenda's infection had been brought on by her diabetes, her "careless" health habits, and her active sexual history.

Robins-Zelle attorneys knew that A. H. Robins would attack Brenda's character, for it had become part of the company's standard defense in recent years. Ciresi called it A. H. Robins' "three-dog defense." First the company would try to prove that the Shield was not a defective device. But in case the jury wasn't willing to buy that, A. H. Robins would argue that even if the Shield created a health risk to women, the risk was no greater than with any other IUD. And finally, just for extra protection, they would go after the woman, attacking her character, inquiring into the most intimate and usually irrelevant details of her sexual life, implying that she had somehow "dirtied" herself and thus was to blame for her infection.

These questions, which quickly became known as A. H. Robins' "Dirty Questions," included:

- At what age did you first become sexually active?
- Did you have any problem achieving orgasm prior to the time the Dalkon Shield was inserted?
- When you go to the bathroom do you wipe from front to back or back to front?
- Do you engage in oral intercourse, and with what frequency?
- Do you use marital aids, such as vibrators and artificial penises?
- Do you engage in intercourse during the time you are menstruating?

They also often asked for the name of every sexual partner the woman had ever had, even those she had prior to her use of the Shield.

One Iowa woman, in her husband's presence, was asked to name her sexual partners prior to her 1963 marriage, which was some 10 years before she received her Dalkon Shield and 15 years before she contracted PID.

This type of questioning had a chilling effect on women filing suits. Many dropped their suits or rushed to an early settlement because they were embarrassed by such private questions and didn't want to be forced to answer them in a public courtroom.

A. H. Robins usually didn't ask these questions of the women in court, but the fact that the women had to answer the questions in depositions before going to trial was often enough to intimidate them. And the women had no way of knowing beforehand which questions would be asked in the open courtroom and which ones wouldn't be. Some of the women's attorneys tried to protect them by offering to answer the questions in writing rather than in the presence of lawyers and court reporters. But A. H. Robins insisted that the women sit in the room and answer the questions out loud.

Just how ridiculous these questions sometimes became can be seen in an exchange between one woman and an A. H. Robins attorney.

"Do you wear pantyhose?" the attorney asked. Previously the attorney had been inquiring into such things as which way the woman wiped, whether she engaged in oral or anal intercourse, and whether she used vibrators—the standard "Dirty Questions."

The woman said yes, she did wear pantyhose.

"Would the pantyhose that you use have a cotton crotch, or would they be nylon from top to bottom?" the attorney continued.

"I'll answer that," said the woman, "but this sounds more like an obscene phone call than anything else."

A. H. Robins had no evidence that using a particular type of pantyhose would lead to pelvic infection (nor is there such evidence), yet its attorney felt free to question the woman about her pantyhose preferences.

Nor, as a judge later noted, has A. H. Robins ever "come forth with any compelling reason for, or expert testimony supporting, inquiry into which way a person wiped, the use of marital aides, the methods of sexual practice, or whether a woman did not or did achieve orgasm are relevant to what caused her pelvic infection. Not one of [A. H. Robins'] expert witnesses in any trial has ever stated that these 'risk factors' which are 'associated' with pelvic infection caused a particular plaintiff's PID." Yet the company continued to harass and embarrass women with these questions.

To understand why these and other such questions are irrelevant, it must be remembered that the fact that bacteria can be found in the vagina is not the issue. Every woman has some bacteria in her vagina. The bacteria may have entered through intercourse, or on her own hands as she inserted a diaphragm, or even on an artificial penis. The vagina is not supposed to be a sterile place.

But most bacteria that enters the vagina do not migrate on their own into the uterus to cause PID. They usually need help—like a convenient tail string on which to climb. And even if one of these bacteria should enter the uterus during isolated times (such as during the insertion of an IUD), it is usually rendered harmless by the body's natural defense system. Continual entry, however (such as through a tail string), can overload and weaken the defense system, resulting in infection.

There are two organisms that do spread readily from the vagina without help: the gonorrhea bacteria, "gonococcus," and an organism that is a cross between a virus and a bacteria, "chlamydiae." Indeed, before IUDs became widely used in the late 1960s and early 1970s, almost all cases of PID seen by doctors were gonorrhea-related. (Many of these were probably also caused by chlamydiae, but that organism wasn't isolated and identified until the late 1970s.)

Doctors were slow to accept the connection between PID and IUDs. For several years after IUD-related PID was identified, many doctors would continue to write "gonorrhea" on the medical chart of a patient with PID, even when a test for gonorrhea showed up negative. In about 20 percent of gonorrhea tests, women with gonorrhea will "test negative." Thus, many doctors, long used to attributing PID to gonorrhea, would assume gonorrhea was the cause of a woman's PID, even when tests showed no evidence of gonococcus bacteria in her vagina.

This had a devastating effect on many couples' relationships. Either the man would accuse the woman of contracting the "gonorrhea" through an affair, or the woman, knowing she had been faithful, would suspect the man of the same.

A. H. Robins has argued that it needs to question a woman about all her sexual partners to find out if any of them ever had a venereal disease—even if the woman's own medical records show no evidence whatsoever that she ever had the disease herself. In one case in which A. H. Robins attorneys wanted a woman to name all the men, other than her husband, that she had ever slept with, a judge asked the attorneys to show cause why that line of questioning was relevant to the woman's injuries.

"The only way we can find out whether there is a possibility of this woman contracting chlamydiae is to find out about her social history," the attorney said.

A possibility of chlamydiae. A. H. Robins' attorneys had no evidence that she had ever contracted the organism. They wanted to invade her privacy simply on the chance that she had. The judge ruled they could not ask such questions on such a "speculative assertion."

Not all judges have disallowed such questioning and not all doctors think it is necessarily irrelevant. The more sexual partners a woman has, say these doctors, the greater her chances of being exposed to either gonorrhea or chlamydiae. The diseases are almost always active—and therefore test positive—in men, and that is why A. H. Robins argues that it should be able to track down and question all of the men a woman has had intercourse with.

If one of the men is found to have had gonorrhea or chlamydiae, then A. H. Robins can argue that the woman was exposed to the diseases, even if tests show she doesn't have them. This, of course, puts a woman in the impossible position of having to prove a negative. In other words, A. H. Robins does not have to prove that the woman had one of the diseases; the woman must prove that she didn't. Some judges have refused to put women in this position. For even if A. H. Robins were to find that a past sexual partner had gonorrhea or chlamydiae, it "would not tend to produce any relevant evidence which will link the [woman] with the disease," said one judge in a ruling prohibiting the asking of the "Dirty Questions."

Yet another judge has ruled that while a woman's sexual history might have some "marginal relevance," the woman's right to privacy far outweighed A. H. Robins' interest in the matter. The judge also was concerned about the rights of the men involved. "It does not take a great deal of speculation to imagine that some or all of these persons may now be married with families," the judge said. "To permit Robins to discover their identities would be to allow Robins to intrude into their private lives."

Other judges, however, have continued to allow A. H. Robins to track down former sexual partners and ask them detailed questions about their sexual activity of years past—sometimes as many as 15 years past.

In Brenda's trial, the most personal aspects of her life were revealed in open court. The number of lovers she had had before her marriage, an abortion early in her life, a later miscarriage—all came out during the trial and were reported in the local press. These were very private matters for her, matters she had previously kept hidden even from her family. Her mother found out about her abortion after reading about it in the newspaper.

A. H. Robins was relentless. At one point, it became clear to Ciresi that the A. H. Robins' attorneys were going to try to hint to the jury that Brenda had purposely tried to miscarry her baby by not eating or generally taking care of herself. Ciresi jumped up and asked Judge Alsop if counsel for both sides could approach the bench.

Ciresi complained to the judge about where he thought A. H. Robins' attorneys were trying to go with their line of questioning and argued that it had no basis in fact.

"You don't know what they're trying to do," the judge responded.

But the A. H. Robins' attorney confirmed Ciresi's suspicions. "Yep, that's where I'm going," he said.

"No you're not, I'll tell you that right now," the judge said, and that line of questioning ended.

While A. H. Robins' attorneys were going after Brenda, Robins-Zelle attorneys went after the medical experts and medical studies A. H. Robins brought before the jury to show the Shield was no worse than any other device. Robins-Zelle picked the studies apart, one by one.

One of the studies A. H. Robins brought up in the courtroom, for example, had been conducted in England in 1981 under the supervision of Robert Snowden, a sociologist and director of the Institute of Populations Studies at the University of Exeter. The study was based on questionnaires Snowden had sent to doctors at various English clinics asking them about their experiences with IUDs. A. H. Robins asked Snowden to take a retrospective look at the survey forms to see how the Dalkon Shield compared to other IUDs in respect to infections. After this retrospective look, Snowden concluded that the Shield presented no greater danger of PID than any other IUD. In 1976, however, when the survey was first completed, he had told a medical symposium of doctors that the Shield did have a higher incidence of PID than the Copper-7.

There was a box on Snowden's questionnaires for doctors to check if their IUD patients had experienced PID. But Snowden didn't rely on those checked or unchecked boxes in his final analysis for A. H. Robins. Instead, he and his co-researchers went back through all the reports from the doctors to decide themselves what was PID and what wasn't. Ciresi, and others who have looked closely at Snowden's study, claim his criteria for what was PID was too broad. For example, if a doctor indicated that a woman had been put on antibiotics, these critics say, Snowden would mark it down as PID—although the antibiotics might have been prescribed for something that had nothing whatever to do with PID, such as an ear infection. Despite these and other serious questions about Snowden's study, A. H. Robins continues to this day to use the study as its first line of defense when claiming the Shield is no more dangerous with regard to PID than any other IUD.

Brenda's trial lasted three long months. Eighteen expert witnesses were heard; hundreds of documents were discussed. During the trial one juror got married; another died.

Also during the trial, the Centers for Disease Control issued a report urging any woman still wearing a Dalkon Shield to have it removed because it offered a five-times greater risk than other IUDs of leading to PID. The CDC study was based on re-evaluating data collected in the late 1970s from 622 women hospitalized with PID and 2,369 "hospitalized control subjects" with no history of PID—data that was known as the Women's Health Study. The CDC study, published in the July 1983 issue of the *American Journal of Obstetrics & Gynecology,* said that "only 10% of women wearing an IUD were using the Dalkon Shield, yet they accounted for almost 20% of the excess risk of pelvic inflammatory disease occurring among all the IUD users." Ironically, the original conclusion of the Women's Health Study, published in the same medical journal two years earlier, had been that the risk of getting PID was about the same with all IUDs.

The 1983 CDC study said the original study did not discover the increased PID danger presented by the Shield because its authors "did not fully analyze the data by individual IUD type. To determine if the risk of pelvic inflammatory disease varied for the different IUD types, the present authors further analyzed data from the Women's Health Study. It was found that, compared with users of other types of IUDs, women using the Dalkon Shield had a substantially increased risk of pelvic inflammatory disease requiring hospitalization."

During the final week of the trial, Brenda, who had been trying for several years to get pregnant, was told by her doctor that a pregnancy test had shown up positive. For Ciresi and Larson, it was terrible timing, the jury might not be inclined to award a pregnant woman as much money as they would if she were sterile. Ciresi and Larson asked the judge to delay the trial for two weeks until Brenda's pregnancy could indeed be verified. Judge Alsop denied the delay. A. H. Robins' attorneys were notified of Brenda's possible pregnancy—and so was the jury.

In the end, however, it apparently didn't matter. For on June 6, 1983, the jury awarded Brenda $1.75 million dollars for her Dalkon Shield injuries. Only $250,000 was in compensatory damages; the rest of the award was for punitive damages.

The eight-member jury had decided that the Dalkon Shield was defectively designed and manufactured and inadequately tested, and that A. H. Robins had failed to warn doctors of its risks. They awarded the punitive damages to punish A. H. Robins for "willful and indifferent conduct."

It was quite a victory for Robins-Zelle. For Brenda, however, the joy of winning her case was soon overshadowed by the news that the pregnancy test was in error; she was not pregnant.

Within months, Ciresi and Larson were back in a Minnesota courtroom fighting yet another Dalkon Shield battle. They won that one, too.

A. H. Robins suddenly had a formidable opponent on its hands. But the company's problems in Minnesota were just beginning. In another Twin Cities courtroom a federal judge known for his "prairie justice" was about to enter the fray.

A. H. Robins was about to learn just how cold Minnesota could be.

18

Lord Speaks

"Thou shall not steal applies to every corporate official who sells shoddy, dangerous, or unusable merchandise in the name of profit. Thou shall not kill applies to the corporations and agencies of those who are killing and maiming through industrial pollution. This is done by individuals, by corporate leaders who must some day appear in somebody's church. They should appear with the same attitude of contrition and humility which accompanies every other sin."
—U.S. District Judge Miles Lord, in a speech
before the Minnesota Council of Churches, 1981.

When U.S. District Judge Miles Lord was assigned 23 Dalkon Shield cases in December 1983, he had no idea that these cases would lead him into the biggest controversy of his already spirited and controversial career.

Within nine months, Lord would find himself standing before five of his fellow federal judges, accused of judicial misconduct for sharply reprimanding three A. H. Robins executives in his courtroom. The accusation would land him a segment on "60 Minutes" and the notice of columnists and editorial writers across the country.

But then controversy was not new to Miles Lord. In 1980, *The American Lawyer*, a legal trade magazine, named him the worst judge in the 8th Circuit and one of the 11 worst in the country. The following year, the Association of Trial Lawyers of America honored Lord as the outstanding federal judge of the year.

Lord is not a judge who engenders indifferent or neutral opinions. His critics called him a "judicial gadfly," a "grandstander," a judge who improperly picks sides in the cases before him and therefore plays the role of an advocate rather than of a neutral observer. His supporters call him a champion of the underdog, a smart and effective judge who is able to cut through legal brambles and get to the heart—and justice—of even the most complicated of cases.

Few doubt that Lord's aggressive effort to find the truth in the Dalkon Shield saga dramatically changed the course of future litigation. Indeed, he was the first judge to attack A. H. Robins' behavior openly and finally break through the company's carefully constructed shield of defense.

Lord is often described by friends and foes alike as "the last of the prairie populist judges." Former Vice President Hubert H. Humphrey, Lord's close friend and the man responsible for getting him appointed to the federal court, called Lord "a people's judge." Certainly, Lord's history is rooted in Minnesota's rural communities, if not technically on its prairies. He was born in 1919 on a small and impoverished farm on Minnesota's "Iron Range," a taconite mining area near the center of the state. His father was a logger; his mother, a Sunday school teacher. Lord was their eighth child.

A Golden Gloves middleweight boxer and jitterbug champion, Lord worked his way through the University of Minnesota with a host of odd jobs, including part-time janitor, night watchman, bellhop, postal clerk, and welder. After getting his law degree, he made a bid for a seat in the Minnesota State House. He lost that race, but went on to become assistant U.S. attorney, where he made a name for himself by prosecuting racketeers around Minneapolis. But he found politics suited his gregarious nature, and eventually was elected the state's attorney general. Later he was appointed U.S. attorney for Minnesota and then, in 1966, President Lyndon Johnson named him to the federal bench.

Lord has never hidden his impatience with an American society that appears to him to treat corporate wrongdoers differently than other lawbreakers.

"If the corporate officers direct their corporation into violating the law to make profit, and they are caught and pay a fine, that's looked upon as a nuisance, a nonrecurring obligation it says in the books, and an unfortunate incursion by outsiders," Lord has said. "The corporate official, the individual who is caught with his fingers in the pie and making antitrust arrangements, polluting, or making unsafe goods, or other arrangements which are contrary to the law, suffers almost no disgrace either in the eyes of his corporate officials and employers, nor the public at large, but rather his conduct is looked upon as being the norm."

Well, Lord made it clear that in his courtroom at least, such activity would not be looked upon as the norm. This attitude has occasionally gotten him into trouble with some of his judicial peers, most notably in the Reserve Mining Company case, which he presided over in the mid-1970s. The case was a precedent of a kind for what happened later with the Dalkon Shield.

In 1974, Lord shut down Reserve's huge taconite plant on Lake Superior because he believed that the 67,000 tons of taconite waste it was dumping into the lake daily, and the pollution from the plant's smokestacks, presented a serious health risk. "The defendants [Reserve] are daily endangering the lives of thousands of people. . . . This Court cannot honor profit over human life and therefore has no other choice but to abate the discharge," Lord ruled.

Within 48 hours, an appeals court overturned Lord's ruling, telling the company instead that it could keep its plant open while it negotiated an alternative dump site for the taconite waste with the state of Minnesota. It also told Lord to stay out of the negotiations. But after negotiations dragged on for two more years—with the waste still being spilled into Lake Superior—Lord violated the order by calling hearings to investigate the delay.

In those hearings, Lord challenged Reserve's credibility and ordered the company to pay $100,000 for the city of Duluth's water filtration system. "I have dispensed with the usual adversary proceeding here," Lord said, "because I simply do not have time to spend, as I did, nine months in hearing, six months of which was wasted by what I find now . . . to be misrepresentations by Reserve Mining Company."

Shortly afterward, the 8th U.S. Circuit Court of Appeals removed Lord from the case because of what it described as his "gross bias" against Reserve and his disregard "for the mandate" of the appellate court, which had told him not to become involved in the site selection. But in the end, Lord was vindicated. The judge who took over the case from him fined Reserve $1 million and charged the company with withholding important evidence from opposing attorneys and from Lord. The dumping of taconite wastes into Lake Superior was finally stopped.

So it was not out of character when, seven years later, Lord reviewed the Dalkon Shield cases assigned to his court and concluded that he needed to cut through the legal thicket and get things moving. Some of the 23 Dalkon Shield cases assigned to him had been pending in court for almost three years.

To speed things up, Lord decided to take the unusual step of consolidating all the cases for one trial and convening a jury of 28 people. This expanded jury would first decide the question of liability; in other words, was A. H. Robins negligent? Then the jurors would be split into three groups to decide, case by case, if the Shield caused the women's specific injuries and, if so, how much each woman should be compensated. When all of the cases were concluded, the jurors would then join together and decide whether A. H. Robins should pay punitive damages as well.

A. H. Robins' lawyers didn't like this idea. They wanted each of the 100 Dalkon Shield cases pending before Minnesota courts and the more than 3,000 then pending nationwide to be tried individually. A. H. Robins knew how a group of consolidated cases would look to a jury: 23 different women with 23 different medical histories. A. H. Robins would have to convince the jury that a whole host of factors could lead to PID— for example, diabetes in one woman, an elective abortion in another, and an active sexual history in yet another. At the same time A. H. Robins would have to try to convince the jury that the Shield hadn't caused PID in any of the women, that this wasn't an epidemic. "When you can get a cross section of eight or ten women, [Robins] is dead in the water," says Robins-Zelle attorney Roger Brosnahan. "Then the only common factor to all of those women and their problems is the Dalkon Shield."

Lord announced his decision to consolidate the cases in a December 9, 1983, meeting with attorneys from both sides. He also said that he wasn't going to go through the kind of protracted document struggle that occurred in earlier Shield cases. If a document had been accepted into evidence by another judge, it would be accepted in his courtroom.

At that meeting Lord also announced his decision to reopen the discovery process. This was a major step. Previously, discovery in the Shield cases had been allowed only twice—in the mid-1970s after the cases were brought under the Multi-District Litigation (MDL) process, and again in 1982, when the judge overseeing the MDL had permitted plaintiffs' attorneys to request more documents from A. H. Robins. Since then, however, the discovery door had been shut. Now Lord was permitting attorneys representing the women to look for still more documents and, even more significantly, to talk with A. H. Robins' top officials about what they knew and when they knew it. Attorneys from Robins-Zelle, who had been appointed lead counsel for the women plaintiffs, were obviously excited. They would finally have a chance to question A. H. Robins' top officials.

The depositions began in January 1984. The stories A. H. Robins' top officials told in those depositions were remarkable. One by one, the officials claimed no knowledge of, nor any responsibility for, the Dalkon Shield tragedy.

E. Claiborne Robins, Jr., president of A. H. Robins since 1978, testified that he did not know if anyone in A. H. Robins' management from a division head up had ever evaluated the Dalkon Shield situation or discussed it with outside consultants. Yet he acknowledged that "the Dalkon Shield has always been a concern to A. H. Robins" and that "the future of our company can be affected by the Dalkon Shield litigation." Why a president of a company would not ask his managers if they had reviewed a situation that might direly affect the future of the company (not to mention the health of millions of women) seems puzzling at best.

Dr. Carl Lunsford, head of A. H. Robins' research and development division since the mid-1970s and the man responsible for the safety and efficacy of all A. H. Robins' medical products, also appeared surprisingly disinterested in the Dalkon Shield. Although acknowledging that he knew the Shield's tail string could wick bacteria, Lunsford testified that he had never talked to anyone in A. H. Robins' medical department about how this wicking might affect a woman's uterus. As far as he knew, he said, no one at A. H. Robins knew how a multifilament string works or what happens to it in the uterus—and he had never felt it necessary to ask someone to find out. As a manager, Lunsford seems to have been remarkably lax. Fletcher Owen, the man A. H. Robins says has been "monitoring" the Shield since it was taken off the market, was Lunsford's responsibility; Owen reported directly to him. Yet Lunsford testified that he did not know what Owen was doing to monitor the Shield. Nor had he ever asked Owen whether he had received any reports from doctors about problems with the Shield.

But perhaps the most remarkable statement coming from this man whose job it is to check A. H. Robins' products for safety is that he has never once asked any A. H. Robins employee or consultant if the Shield was unsafe. Not once.

No one, it would seem, talks about the Dalkon Shield at A. H. Robins. It's as if it never existed, as if it were just the figment of 2.4 million women's imaginations.

Indeed, passing the buck seems to have reached new heights at A. H. Robins, as Judge Frank Theis, the Wichita judge who presided over the discovery process during the MDL proceedings, has noted. "The project manager for Dalkon Shield explains that a particular question should have gone to the medical department, the medical department representative explains that the question was really the bailiwick of the quality control department, and the quality control department representative explains that the project manager was the one with the authority to make a decision on that question," Theis wrote. With such a denial of responsibility, the judge noted, "it is not at all unusual for the hard questions posed in Dalkon Shield cases to be unanswerable by anyone from Robins."

The taking of the depositions of A. H. Robins' top officials progressed very slowly during that winter of 1984. The officials' answers to questions were often vague and noncommittal. "I don't recall" became a common answer, even to the most basic questions.

This was especially true of E. Claiborne Robins, Sr.'s deposition. He said he could not recall any conversations with A. H. Robins' top officials regarding the Dalkon Shield. When asked if the minutes of the company's board of directors meetings would help refresh his memory, he said yes. A. H. Robins' attorneys, however, refused to provide those minutes.

On January 23, 1984, frustrated Robins-Zelle attorneys called Judge Lord and told him of the stalled deposition. Lord ordered A. H. Robins to produce the board meeting minutes to aid its chairman's memory. A. H. Robins' attorneys, however, turned over only excerpts of the minutes. They claimed that some of the references to the Shield that appeared in the minutes was the privileged information of attorney and client.

Lord told A. H. Robins he would decide what was privileged and what was not. He ordered the attorneys to bring the minute books to Minneapolis for his review. On January 25, Lord sat in his chambers with A. H. Robins' attorney Alexander Slaughter on one side and Robins-Zelle attorney Roger Brosnahan on the other.

"And the judge is looking through the minutes of five years . . . and he says, 'There's stuff in here that's relevant. There's stuff in here that's impeaching. There's stuff in here that [calls for] sanctions,'" recalls Brosnahan. "He was furious. When he saw those minutes and saw what those people were told at monthly meetings, he said, 'We're going to get the truth out of them.'" By "impeaching," the judge meant that the material challenged the credibility of A. H. Robins' officials. By saying it called for sanctions, he meant it was serious enough that the court could take some actions against those officials.

What the minutes revealed, Lord later wrote, was that "both Robins Sr. and his son, Chief Executive Officer E. C. Robins, Jr., not only attended nearly every board meeting during their tenures in office but also demonstrated a detailed knowledge of the corporation's affairs. These were crucial revelations, given the fact that both of these officers claimed lack of knowledge due to both poor recollection of events and limited participation in the concerns of the company." After reading the minutes

Lord believed that there probably existed other documents relevant to the Dalkon Shield—documents that had not been produced during the MDL discovery.

The next day Lord was in Richmond, personally supervising the depositions and the discovery process. He didn't like what he saw.

"The scene in Richmond . . . was far from conducive to orderly court proceedings," the judge later wrote. "The depositions of Robins Sr. and [retired] company officer Dr. Fred A. Clark Jr. were being conducted at the company's insistence in its own headquarters. Company employees milled about, leaving plaintiffs' attorneys no privacy in which to confer with each other. Live microphones further intruded on any discussions between the plaintiffs' attorneys. Chairs were positioned so that attorneys for the deponents [Robins' officials] sat shoulder-to-shoulder, knee-to-knee with their clients; a nudge by an attorney could—and did—silence the deponent without anyone else in the room picking up the signal. The deposition room itself was small and poorly ventilated. Heat from lights used to videotape the depositions raised the room's temperature to more than 80 degrees."

Lord suggested to A. H. Robins' attorneys that the proceedings be moved to a more comfortable site at the Richmond courthouse, but the attorneys objected. (Yet they had earlier tried to prevent two A. H. Robins' officials, E. Claiborne, Sr., and Fred Clark, from testifying, claiming the men were suffering from heart disease. Certainly, the heat in those cramped rooms was not conducive to their good health. Although they had agreed to the visit earlier, halfway through Lord's planned two-day trip to Richmond, A. H. Robins' attorneys objected to his being present. He flew back to Minneapolis, where discovery again progressed at a snail's pace.

A. H. Robins fought every request for new document production. To make its arguments, the company sent an ever-shifting team of attorneys into Lord's courtroom, a practice that severely tried Lord's patience. Lord accepted A. H. Robins' need for a large legal team, given the high stakes involved. "However, what is absolutely unacceptable is the defendant's practice of obscuring the responsibility of its attorneys so that it is impossible to determine at any given moment who is accountable for representations made to the court," Lord later wrote. "[Robins] also has rotated its attorneys in and out so that the court must start up from ground level over and over in order to brief the new arrival."

At one point, for example, a Minneapolis attorney that A. H. Robins had hired to work with its Richmond attorneys on the case submitted a legal brief to Judge Lord which Lord thought was inaccurate. When he asked about the inaccuracies, the local attorney was unable to defend them, for he had never read the documents covered in the brief. Indeed, when Lord asked him who had written the brief, the attorney answered, "I'm not real sure, your Honor." The brief had been prepared in Richmond, then sent to Minneapolis for the attorney to present to the court.

Judge Lord wasn't the first judge who had become angered by these "shell game tactics" of A. H. Robins. A Florida judge had earlier criticized the company for the same tactics. Lord, however, decided to do something about it, to put an end to this "parade of defense attorneys," few of whom seemed to have the knowledge or the authority to answer Lord's questions. Lord demanded that each person who worked on a document sign it before submitting it to the court and that each out-of-town lawyer sign an oath promising to abide by and be subject to the same rules of ethics as all Minnesota attorneys.

A. H. Robins' attorneys were outraged. They considered Lord's demand an attack on their integrity and refused to sign the oaths. Lord and the attorneys battled over the oath for several days, finally settling on a watered-down version. It was also agreed that each brief or document submitted to the court would be signed by the attorneys who had worked on it.

While the argument over the production of documents continued, Lord was deciding other issues pertinent to the consolidated cases before him. He had been incensed by the kind of questioning that had gone on in Brenda's trial a year earlier. He told A. H. Robins' attorneys that before he would allow them to ask personal questions of the women, A. H. Robins would have to show that the subject of the question "caused or contributed" to the woman's injuries.

On February 8, 1984, exasperated by A. H. Robins' attempts to hinder the discovery process, Lord issued an order that had a profound and lasting effect on Dalkon Shield litigation. He ordered A. H. Robins to produce thousands of new documents in 10 categories he carefully detailed. He also appointed two special court masters to weed through the documents and to decide which were privileged and which should be made available to attorneys representing the women.

(A year later, these two masters, after going through all the new documents, wrote a report to the U.S. District Court in Minnesota highly critical of A. H. Robins. "We conclude that plaintiffs have established a strong prima facie case that A. H. Robins Co., Inc. has, with the knowledge and participation of in-house counsel, engaged in an ongoing fraud by knowingly misrepresenting the nature, quality, safety and efficacy of the Dalkon Shield," the masters wrote. "The ongoing fraud has also involved the destruction or withholding of relevant evidence.")

The next day, A. H. Robins' attorneys appealed Lord's order to the 8th Circuit Court of Appeals. A few days later, the company filed a motion asking Lord to remove himself from the case because of an "unprecedented degree of hostility and bias toward Robins. . . . In short, the trial judge has put on a cloak of partiality and has injected himself into the proceedings not as an unbiased arbiter, but as a partisan advocate."

Lord had heard words like that before, in the Reserve Mining case; but now, as then, he felt his actions were justified. "As the arguments against production of the documents exhaust themselves, the tribunal itself becomes the target," he wrote in response. "This court has tasted of this cup before; it has had its fill."

Lord did not step down from the case, and on February 23, 1984, the appeals court upheld his document production order. By now, only two of the original 23 Dalkon Shield cases remained to be tried before Judge Lord. A. H. Robins' attorneys, uneasy over Lord's reopening of the discovery process, had been gradually settling the cases since January, making offers that the women and Robins-Zelle attorneys could not refuse. Now, having lost their appeal to a higher court, they were even more anxious to get out of Lord's courtroom—and thus out from under his order for more documents. Furthermore, they had no intention of coming back. The company had made sure of that by hiring as part of its local defense team the St. Paul law firm where Judge Lord's son-in-law worked. Judicial ethics demanded that Lord disqualify himself from any future Shield cases assigned to him.

Robins-Zelle attorneys, on the other hand, wanted to hold off settlement on the last two cases for as long as possible. Every day the cases remained open meant more documents could be unearthed by the special masters, who were working feverishly in Richmond. Those documents would prove useful in the 300 other suits Robins-Zelle had pending against A. H. Robins.

The race was on, and it finally came to an end on February 29, 1984. A. H. Robins agreed to pay $4.6 million to settle the two cases and five other cases represented by Robins-Zelle. This was more money than Robins-Zelle had originally asked for.

A. H. Robins made other concessions as well. They agreed not to try to transfer Minnesota cases to out-of-state courts, something it had attempted previously. They agreed to itemize and preserve the documents Lord had ordered produced in a special library in Richmond. Those documents that A. H. Robins agreed were not privileged would be made available to Robins-Zelle attorneys at the library; those documents the company claimed were privileged would be presented to a judge for a ruling.

It seemed, then, that Judge Lord had succeeded in his original goal to get the 23 cases before him settled quickly and justly. But Lord wondered if justice had truly been served. To Lord, the provisions of the settlement seemed to benefit only the women represented by Robins-Zelle—and put an end to the discovery process in Richmond.

Most disturbing to Lord, however, was the fact that A. H. Robins' top executives had not had to face up to what their company had done. Lord wanted them at least to acknowledge the years of suffering by women who had been injured by the Shield. He also wanted them to keep the document production open and to recall the Shield.

To make sure the executives could no longer hide behind a mask of ignorance, Lord asked three A. H. Robins officials—E. Claiborne Robins, Sr., William Forrest, and Fred Clark—to attend the settlement hearing on Wednesday, February 29. But it was a demand by Robins-Zelle that the three be present as a condition of settlement, that got the officials on the plane to Minneapolis. (Attorneys for Robins, Sr., and Clark said they were too ill to attend the hearing, so E. Claiborne, Jr., and Carl Lunsford came in their place.)

Knowing the officers would be present, Lord prepared a statement the previous weekend. Lord says he initially intended to deliver his remarks to the three officers as a private reprimand. Indeed, when the officers appeared in his courtroom that Monday morning, he first had them read the statement silently to themselves. But when he attempted to ask them afterward if his speech had had any impact on them, attorneys for the officials rose up and told their clients not to answer.

Lord was angered by what he later referred to as the officials' "undisguised disdain for the Court." If the men would not be chastised privately, then he would do it publicly. So, for nearly half an hour, he read the statement aloud in open court. The three officers sat silently before him as he read; only Lunsford looked uneasy, anxious to be somewhere else.

"It is not enough to say, 'I did not know,' 'It was not me,' 'Look elsewhere,'" Lord began. "Time and time again, each of you has used this kind of argument in refusing to acknowledge your responsibility and in pretending to the world that the chief officers and the directors of your gigantic multinational corporation have no responsibility for the company's acts and omissions. . . .

"Today as you sit here attempting once more to extricate yourselves from the legal consequences of your acts, none of you has faced up to the fact that more than 9,000 women have made claims that they gave up part of their womanhood so that your company might prosper. It is alleged that others gave their lives so you might so prosper. And there stand behind them legions more who have been injured but who have not sought relief in the courts of this land.

"I dread to think what would have been the consequences if your victims had been men rather than women, women who seem through some strange quirk of our society's mores to be expected to suffer pain, shame and humiliation.

"If one poor young man were by some act of his—without authority or consent—to inflict such damage upon one woman, he would be jailed for a good portion of the rest of his life. And yet your company, without warning to women, invaded their bodies by the millions and caused them injuries by the thousands. And when the time came for these women to make their claims against your company, you attacked their characters. You inquired into their sexual practices and into the identity of their sex partners. You exposed these women—and ruined families and reputations and careers—in order to intimidate those who would raise their voices against you. You introduced issues that had no relationship whatsoever to the fact that you planted in the bodies of these women instruments of death, of mutilation, of disease."

Lord continued reading, slowly, deliberately, in the silent courtroom. He pleaded with the three men to stop the "monstrous mischief" of their company and to recall the Shield.

"If this were a case in equity, I would order that your company make an effort to locate each and every woman who still wears this device and recall your product. But this court does not have the power to do so. I must therefore resort to moral persuasion and a personal appeal to each of you. . . . You've got lives out there, people, women, wives, moms, and some who will never be moms. . . . You are the corporate conscience. Please, in the name of humanity, lift your eyes above the bottom line."

When Lord had finished reading, an A. H. Robins attorney jumped up and objected strongly to the judge's remarks. "You have become an advocate for the plaintiffs' position," he said.

"I certainly have," Lord answered. "At the end of this case, after reviewing thousands of documents, looking at the briefs, reading the depositions . . . I have concluded that the plaintiffs are right and that the things I say are based—they are my judgments based on the record. . . . You don't have to argue that I am prejudiced at this point. I am."

Cynthia Parker, the Minnesota woman who had lost her baby after becoming pregnant while wearing the Shield, was in the courtroom that day, sitting in a back row among the attorneys and reporters. Hers had not been one of the cases before Judge Lord, but when she had heard that A. H. Robins officials would be in Lord's courtroom that day, she had felt a need to be there, to see them face to face. As Lord read his statement, tears had come to Cynthia's eyes. Finally someone was telling the A. H. Robins officials what Cynthia had wanted to tell them for years.

But A. H. Robins' officials apparently did not hear what Lord and Cynthia had hoped they would hear. In a bitter speech at the A. H. Robins' annual meeting a few weeks later, E. Claiborne, Jr., charged that Lord's speech was nothing more than a "poisonous attack upon this company, its people and its product."

Point by point, he countered Lord's allegations. "[Lord] formed the opinion that the Dalkon Shield is dangerously defective without hearing a word of expert medical testimony," he said. "A. H. Robins' position is that the greater weight of the medical evidence shows that the infection rate associated with the Dalkon Shield is not statistically different from infection associated with other IUDs."

What E. Claiborne, Jr., failed to tell those attending the meeting, however, was that A. H. Robins had paid for many of those favorable studies and that it had kept unfavorable data from public scrutiny.

E. Claiborne, Jr., also lashed out at plaintiffs' attorneys in his speech. "It is my strong belief," he said, "that we are locked in an economic battle with the plaintiffs' bar which is more concerned about how to pick our corporate pocket than it is about righting any alleged wrong related to the Dalkon Shield."

Finally, he charged that Lord had purposively painted a one-toned picture of A. H. Robins. "Judge Lord obviously wasn't looking for good," E. Claiborne, Jr., said. "He wasn't prepared to be impartial, as befits a judge. Instead, he was prepared to destroy, to tear down and to demean. Now, Judge Lord may say that the good deeds of this Company and its leaders have no bearing on the right or wrong of Dalkon Shield litigation. But he chose to question the integrity, the honesty and the compassion of our people. Well, he was wrong."

If A. H. Robins had hoped to stop document production by settling its cases before Judge Lord, it was soon disappointed. Other Minnesota judges followed Lord's lead and ordered A. H. Robins to keep what were now known as the "Judge Lord documents" available in Richmond. Lord's speech also seemed to awaken judges in other states to the fact that A. H. Robins might have been less than forthcoming in Dalkon Shield cases tried in their courts.

In July 1984, Judge Frank Theis in Wichita, the judge who had presided over the MDL discovery, indicated that he now believed he might have been misled. "I was satisfied . . . that all available relevant evidence in the possession of A. H. Robins and its attorneys had been made available," he wrote. "It would appear that representations made to me . . . are open to serious question."

What is in these "new" documents that A. H. Robins has fought so hard to protect? The set of documents that seems to generate the most interest, from attorneys for women and for A. H. Robins, involves lab notebooks and other raw data from a series of Dalkon Shield tail string tests A. H. Robins' attorneys sponsored starting around 1977. Plaintiffs' attorneys have dubbed these the "secret studies." A. H. Robins has gone to great lengths to keep them out of the courtroom. Whenever a judge has ruled that they must be produced, the company suddenly offers settlements that lawyers find impossible to refuse.

A. H. Robins claims the information in these studies is privileged because the studies were instigated at the request of its attorneys and because the results of the studies have never been communicated to the company itself. The studies were never published; the raw data was simply given to A. H. Robins' attorneys, sometimes with a brief written report, sometimes with only an oral explanation of the findings. Attorneys are permitted by law to keep secret any mental impressions they gather while preparing to defend a client. In other words, because the attorneys rather than A. H. Robins' medical department asked for the studies, the company now claims the studies are the work-product of its attorneys and thus can be kept secret.

A. H. Robins has been vague about what is in the studies, although the company has indicated that it believes they show that the Dalkon Shield was no more harmful to women than any other IUD. But one plaintiff's attorney who has seen the data in the studies says A. H. Robins' public evaluation of the data is not accurate. The studies confirm Howard Tatum's studies and clearly show the Shield to be more dangerous than other IUDs, the attorney says.

In fact, the attorney calls one of the notebooks from a 1977 study "devastating" for A. H. Robins. "[The notebook] is probably the single most important piece of information in the entire [Dalkon Shield] litigation," says the attorney.

The mystery surrounding these secret studies has been heightened by some of A. H. Robins' own actions. In the spring of 1984, while all A. H. Robins documents pertaining to the Dalkon Shield were under a judge's protective order that prohibited A. H. Robins from destroying them, boxes of Dalkon Shield papers were removed from the home of a former

A. H. Robins' attorney, Harris Wagenseil. He had been the attorney in charge of setting up the studies for A. H. Robins. Wagenseil said that he had not been notified of the protective order and that his wife had thrown the documents away while housecleaning.

The weekend the documents were thrown away preceded—coincidentally—the Monday on which A. H. Robins had been ordered to turn over a description of the secret studies to Minnesota attorney Patricia Hartmann. She was the first attorney to pursue the studies and to persuade a judge that women injured by the Shield had a compelling need to see the studies—a need that should override the work-product privilege claim of A. H. Robins' attorneys.

Also, one of A. H. Robins' experts and well-paid witnesses, a witness they have used in many trials, was caught giving conflicting testimony about his role in a Robins-instigated tail string study. In a 1983 Florida trial, A. H. Robins called Louis Keith, a Chicago gynecologist, to testify about the Shield's tail string. Under oath, Keith was asked if he had done or was doing any studies under his direction on the Dalkon Shield tail string.

"Yes," Keith testified. "Studies are being done under my direction." Keith went on to state that the general purpose of the experiments was "to gain information on the allegation that had been made by some individuals that the string wicked bacteria." He even drew a diagram in the courtroom to explain the manner in which the experiments were conducted.

But eight months later, in a California case, Dr. Keith gave quite a different testimony.

"Have you done any experimental work on new Dalkon Shield tail strings?" an attorney for a woman asked Keith.

"No, other than to look at one I think under the microscope," Keith replied.

"You haven't done any wicking experiments?"

"I haven't."

"Has somebody under your supervision done some?"

"Not under my supervision. I didn't supervise anybody."

"Has somebody at your request done some wicking experiments?"

Keith responded that he had knowledge that a professor of microbiology at Chicago Medical School had done some.

"When did he do these?" the attorney asked him.

"Within the last six months."

"Are those the same ones that you testified about in Florida?"

"Yes."

But, of course, as an appellate court later pointed out, "he obviously could not have possessed any knowledge" of those experiments for they had not yet been conducted at the time he testified in Florida.

A. H. Robins described the discrepancy in Keith's testimony as "trivial." But the 11th Circuit Court of Appeals saw it otherwise. On January 21, 1985, it declared Keith had committed perjury and ordered a new trial for the Florida woman. And it issued some strong words to A. H. Robins' attorneys:

"Robins states that . . . allegations of attorney complicity are baseless," the ruling noted. "However, in view of the fact that Dr. Keith had acted as a consultant/expert for Robins attorneys since 1977, it becomes obvious that Robins' counsel must have been aware that Dr. Keith's testimony in [California] contradicted his testimony in [Florida] . . . This court is deeply disturbed by the fact that a material expert witness, with complicity of counsel, would falsely testify on the ultimate issue of causation."

On April 19, 1984, Michael Ciresi stood in a room at A. H. Robins' Richmond headquarters taking the deposition of Patricia Lashley, William Forrest's former secretary, who now worked as a paralegal assistant. Two months earlier, Lashley had revealed in the first session of the deposition the existence of two important, and previously unknown, documents: a tape of A. H. Robins' 1974 septic abortion conference and shorthand notes of the 1975 meeting following Connie Deemer's trial in which A. H. Robins officials gathered to discuss what each of them knew about the Dalkon Shield.

The first session of Lashley's deposition had been stopped because of the settlement of the cases in Judge Lord's courtroom. Now it was being resumed for other Robins-Zelle cases. On this day, however, Lashley changed her story, stating that the tape had never existed and that the folder that should contain the shorthand notes was empty.

Ciresi immediately asked that the folder be placed in a cellophane bag and preserved for fingerprinting. The A. H. Robins attorney present with Lashley refused, claiming such an action wasn't part of Lord's discovery order.

"I'll be glad to call Judge Lord right now and ask him if that would be appropriate, if you think it's a violation of his order," said Ciresi.

"Well, I thought Judge Lord excused himself from this litigation," the A. H. Robins attorney responded.

"Well, you're talking about his order, and I'll be glad to call Judge

Lord if you feel it's a violation of his order and get his approval for it," Ciresi said.

Five days later, A. H. Robins filed two complaints against Judge Lord with the 8th Circuit Court of Appeals. The complaints alleged that by calling the three A. H. Robins executives to his courtroom and sternly lecturing them, Lord had "grossly abused his office." The company wanted Lord investigated for misconduct, and it wanted the speech expunged from the record so it could not be used in other trials. Failure to remove it from the record, A. H. Robins argued, would cause the company "immeasurable" harm in thousands of other Dalkon Shield cases.

But Lord and others believed A. H. Robins was really trying to end Lord's jurisdiction over the troublesome document production.

The showdown between Lord and A. H. Robins was a national event. A. H. Robins brought in former U.S. Attorney General Griffin Bell, who described Lord's actions in the Dalkon Shield litigation as "burrs under the saddle . . . [that] need to be removed so we can get on with it." Not to be outdone, Lord brought in former U.S. Attorney General Ramsey Clark, who promptly charged Bell with signing complaints against Lord that contained "serious deceptive statements." Bell argued that Lord, by lecturing the three A. H. Robins officials, had deprived them of their constitutional rights. Clark called Bell's argument "bizarre."

The charges and countercharges between Lord and A. H. Robins finally ended in a draw. Lord was cleared of misconduct charges, but his speech was expunged from the record.

Lord's battle for the truth was personally expensive, however. His integrity had been publicly challenged, and privately he was now facing legal bills of $110,000.

Lord's speech may have had little effect on the executives, but it did touch others. Hundreds of women, for the first time, became aware that medical problems they had suffered might have been caused by the Shield. Other women who had been injured by the Shield wrote to Lord thanking him for speaking out on their behalf.

But perhaps the one person most significantly moved by the speech was a law professor at Oral Roberts University in Tulsa, Oklahoma. The speech prompted him to step forward and reveal secrets about the Shield, secrets he had concealed for almost a decade.

Born Again

"Having put my foot on the tar baby it will be hard to extricate it."

—Roger Tuttle, former A. H. Robins attorney, during a break in his deposition, July 1984.

The morning of July 30, 1984, was one of expectation in U.S. District Judge Earl Cudd's Minneapolis courtroom.

In the witness chair sat Roger Tuttle, the bespectacled and unimposing law professor from Oral Roberts University, the man who had once managed A. H. Robins' Dalkon Shield litigation, the man who might hold the answers to questions women and lawyers had been asking for years about the Dalkon Shield.

Less than a year earlier, Tuttle had infuriated A. H. Robins and delighted attorneys representing women in Dalkon Shield suits by publishing an article in the *Oklahoma Bar Journal*. In the article, entitled "The Dalkon Shield Disaster Ten Years Later—A Historical Perspective," he had reviewed the Dalkon Shield story, and had come to some conclusions that strongly suggested A. H. Robins' role in the drama had been less than honorable.

"Robins entered a therapeutic area with no prior experience, no trained personnel, and reliance on statistics from an admittedly biased source," Tuttle wrote. "Although the device was based on sound scientific principles, Robins over promoted it without doing sufficient clinical testing in an effort to ride the crest of a marketing wave for financial gain. . . . Robins took advantage of the hiatus in the federal statute between the

214

requirements for clinical trials on drugs and the lack thereof for devices, and marketed a device that looked good in scientific theory but that performed differently in actual practice. Had Robins been willing to wait for the results of its own testing to confirm [Hugh] Davis's results, thus forgoing immediate profit, it likely would not be in the difficult position it faces today."

After the article was published, A. H. Robins criticized Tuttle harshly, claiming he had violated the lawyer's code of professional responsibility. Tuttle said he used only information that was on the public record in his article. He also revealed that he had a letter from William Zimmer "waiving the privilege and excusing me from responsibilities in respect of . . . a broad secrecy agreement that I had executed as a condition precedent to my employment." He said the letter specifically waived any secrecy agreement on the Dalkon Shield.

It was little wonder Tuttle's article made A. H. Robins uneasy. Tuttle was more than just an ex-Robins employee. He was the attorney who, during most of his five years with the company, had been in charge of defending the Dalkon Shield. He knew the players, he'd been to the meetings, and he'd read the memos. Indeed, Tuttle had been A. H. Robins' lead attorney in the disastrous Connie Deemer lawsuit in 1975. For A. H. Robins, the loss of the Deemer case marked the beginning of years of multi-million dollar legal problems. For Tuttle, it marked the effective end of his career with the company.

Tuttle had been an important figure in the Dalkon Shield story, and now he was ready to blow the whistle on his former employer, although no one expected the blast to be as loud as it was.

Michael Ciresi had been trying to get Tuttle's deposition for months. After the *Oklahoma Bar Journal* article, A. H. Robins had sued Tuttle and obtained a temporary restraining order in Oklahoma to prevent the law professor from talking—a restraining order that Tuttle described as being "so broad it had prohibited me from talking to my wife, even." But the restraining order was lifted.

After A. H. Robins realized it was not going to stop Tuttle from talking, the company had tried to at least have the deposition taken in Oklahoma, where Tuttle lived and worked. A. H. Robins did not want the deposition taken in what attorney William Forrest believed to be the "poisoned atmosphere" of Minnesota.

But that effort, too, had failed and on July 30, 1984, nine-and-a-half years after leaving A. H. Robins, Roger Tuttle was in Minneapolis and ready to talk.

A. H. Robins had brought in Thomas H. Sloan, Jr., an attorney with the San Francisco law firm of Bronson, Bronson and McKinnon, to defend its interests during the deposition. Sloan would repeatedly attempt to invoke attorney-client privilege to limit Tuttle's testimony.

Ciresi began with the standard introductions, then asked Tuttle if he'd brought with him, as his subpoena requested, "any documents that you had within your possession which related in any way to your employment or involvement with the A. H. Robins Company and involvement with the Dalkon Shield." Tuttle confirmed that he had two manila envelopes of documents with him, but said that he, as a lawyer, was worried about violating attorney-client privilege.

Sloan didn't miss the opportunity to agree with Tuttle, and stated what was to become his theme for the morning: "Your honor," he said, "I want to make it clear that . . . we [A. H. Robins] are asserting privileges for these documents." The documents were marked into evidence, but not yet into the public record.

Tuttle then ran through his professional background. He graduated from the University of Kansas in 1952, and from the University of Mississippi's law school in 1958. He had a private law practice in Jackson, Mississippi, for several years, then worked several more years as an attorney for the Exxon Corporation in Louisiana and North Carolina. For family reasons, Tuttle said, he left Exxon and moved to Richmond, Virginia, where he spent six years working for an insurance holding company.

In April 1971, based on good recommendations, he was hired at A. H. Robins by Forrest, a man he had met through a Richmond political organization. Tuttle stayed with A. H. Robins for five years, until April 1976, when he left to work for a textile manufacturing firm. He was now a law professor at Oral Roberts University in Tulsa, Oklahoma, where he'd been for the past two-and-a-half years.

Most of the morning's questioning was routine. Tuttle described his responsibilities as a products liability and labor law attorney at A. H. Robins. Part of his job, he said, was to help Forrest review the company's product labeling to make sure it met FDA requirements.

It was pretty innocuous work in the beginning, he said. A. H. Robins had a good reputation, good products, and most of the labeling problems concerned such minor things as moving a symbol from one part of a label to another.

Soon, however, Ciresi's questioning led Tuttle to discuss his frustrations during the Deemer trial. As he prepared for that case, Tuttle said, A. H. Robins' medical department had sandbagged his requests for memos and medical information about the Dalkon Shield. At one point

Tuttle told Ciresi: "I did not receive this [medical] information for so long a period of time that I felt my ability to serve as an attorney was hampered."

Sloan objected repeatedly to Ciresi's questions, but was generally overruled by Judge Cudd.

It was during the afternoon session, however, that Tuttle dropped his "bomb." It came while Ciresi was questioning him about the February 17, 1975, meeting convened by top A. H. Robins officials to discuss the Dalkon Shield; the meeting which Pat Lashley, Forrest's personal secretary, had told Ciresi about in an earlier deposition. Forrest, Zimmer, Freund, Roy Smith, Clark—and Tuttle—had all attended the meeting. Lashley had said she took notes during the meeting, notes that revealed what individual A. H. Robins officials had said they knew about the hazards and characteristics of the Shield. But when Ciresi had requested the folder that those notes had been put in, A. H. Robins attorneys had said it was empty.

"Have you ever seen those stenographic notes of that meeting?" Ciresi asked Tuttle. "No, sir," Tuttle responded after the judge overruled an objection by Sloan. Ciresi tried again, expanding the question: "Have you ever seen transcriptions of any stenographic notes that Ms. Lashley took at any meeting she may have been in attendance at? Regarding the Dalkon Shield, sir."

"I do not believe so," Tuttle said.

Ciresi started another line of questioning for a moment, then stopped. He looked at Tuttle and said: "Have there ever been documents destroyed by A. H. Robins concerning the Dalkon Shield?"

"Yes, sir," Tuttle responded.

The answer caught Ciresi by surprise, as it did others in the courtroom. He quickly looked back toward his legal assistant and raised an eyebrow. "Here we go," he thought to himself.

"When were they destroyed?" Ciresi asked.

Tuttle began sorting through one of the manila envelopes he was holding.

"Excuse me, your honor," Sloan said, "May I halt the proceedings for just a second?" Sloan managed at that time to prevent Tuttle from saying when the documents were destroyed, but it really didn't matter. The damage had been done.

Tuttle's revelation in Cudd's courtroom sent shock waves through law offices across the country. Trying to delay and avoid disclosing documents, as A. H. Robins had done so well in years of Shield litigation, was one thing. Destroying documents was another matter. The documents had not been under a non-destruct order, so the action may not have been illegal. But it certainly raised strong ethical questions and gave credence to Miles Lord's harsh questioning a few months earlier of the moral and ethical nature of A. H. Robins' top officials.

It was Lord's dramatic speech to the A. H. Robins executives, Tuttle said after the deposition, that had convinced him to come forward and reveal the destruction. Tuttle also said he trusted Ciresi to protect him during his deposition from any legal attack from the A. H. Robins attorney. He had given other depositions since leaving A. H. Robins, but had never volunteered the information and had never been asked directly about document destruction.

The destruction, as Tuttle revealed later in his deposition, had taken place in early February 1975, as the jury was deliberating in Connie Deemer's case in Oklahoma.

"Who was involved in the record destruction?" Ciresi asked.

"Well," Tuttle said, "there were persons doing the record search, there was a person who reviewed the records searched, and there were persons who actually physically did the destruction."

Ciresi wanted to know who told the people to destroy the documents. "Pursuant to orders, I did," Tuttle said.

"Who gave you the orders to have documents destroyed?" Ciresi asked. "Mr. Forrest," Tuttle said, referring to A. H. Robins' chief counsel.

Finally, after repeated objections by Sloan, Tuttle named the people who, he said, had actually burned the selected, sensitive documents in a forced-draft furnace at A. H. Robins that was specially designed to destroy contaminated products. The employees actually involved in the search and destroy mission, he said, were Moore; Allen Polon, project coordinator for the Dalkon Shield starting in 1973; Arthur Cummings, an executive assistant in A. H. Robins' international department; Patricia Lashley, Forrest's personal secretary; and Mary Eversole, who was the confidential secretary to George Thomas, a senior vice-president.

Then, seemingly as an afterthought, Tuttle dropped another bombshell on the courtroom: "I might add that not all the . . . documents were actually destroyed."

Tuttle was playing the ace he'd been holding for almost 10 years. "I have documents that were not destroyed," he said, "because I took personal custody of those documents before the other documents were destroyed, and I have preserved them over the years."

Ciresi didn't miss a beat. "Are these documents that bear upon the safety and efficacy of the Dalkon Shield?"

"It's my opinion they do," Tuttle answered.

218

As the afternoon wore on, Tuttle explained that on either February 3 or 4, 1975, Forrest had met with him and ordered the destruction. Did Forrest indicate that he had discussed the destruction with anyone else? "He did," Tuttle said. "Mr. Zimmer."

"Mr. Zimmer was the president of the company at that time?" Ciresi asked. "Yes sir," Tuttle said.

What reason did Forrest give for wanting these documents destroyed, Ciresi asked.

"Mr. Forrest blamed me for the fact that the Clark June 9 memo of 1970 came to light," Tuttle said. (This was the "secret memo" that Post had used to win Connie Deemer's case.)

"His [Forrest's] comments were in words to the effect that he didn't ever want that to happen again, and the only way that it wouldn't happen would be if the documents were no longer in existence," Tuttle said.

Even though there was not a court issued non-destruct order for Dalkon Shield documents at the time, Tuttle said, he was very uneasy about Forrest's order. "It concerned me greatly as an attorney, it concerns me today, that the order was given, that I personally lacked the courage to throw down the gauntlet at that point in time. And that's why I selected out what I considered the most damaging of the documents, some sop for my own conscience as an attorney."

Sloan objected to Tuttle's statement as "non-responsive" and was curtly overruled by Cudd.

Tuttle said he believed the destruction was both morally and legally wrong.

"What was Mr. Forrest's response to your concerns?" Ciresi asked.

"Do it," Tuttle replied. "And I saluted and resisted where I could."

What about the women who had the Shield in their bodies, Ciresi asked. Was there any discussion about them?

"No sir," Tuttle responded.

No discussion at all, Ciresi asked.

"None," Tuttle said. Forrest simply wanted the documents "destroyed and destroyed quickly."

Tuttle described how he sent Moore, Lashley, and the rest of the search crew to pull out Dalkon Shield-related documents from the files of various A. H. Robins executives. With each executive, Tuttle said, "arrangements had to be made and authority given between that individual and Mr. Forrest before I had any right or any of the people who were doing the searching had any right to go in and start going through an executive officer's files."

After documents that A. H. Robins did not want to become public through litigation were removed, the files were returned, he said. The search was extensive and included the files of almost all of A. H. Robins' top officials, Tuttle said. The files of E. C. Robins, Sr., were searched, he said, as were the files of William Zimmer, C. E. Morton, Jack Freund, Roy Smith, and others. Even the files of those doing the searching were searched, Tuttle said.

The files were brought to Tuttle, who reviewed and selected the documents that were damaging or could lead to damaging evidence against A. H. Robins. Those documents, except for the ones he kept, were then tossed in the furnace and burned, he said.

Tuttle was not sure how many documents had been destroyed, but he agreed that it was probably hundreds. A list of the destroyed documents was not kept, Tuttle said, on Forrest's orders.

Tuttle's perception was that his "mandate" for the destruction was to get rid of documents that indicated the "knowledge and complicity, if any, of top officers in the corporation in what at that stage in the game appeared to be a grim situation."

He also said that while the top executives of the company knew their files were being searched by the legal department, Tuttle had no direct indication that they knew Dalkon Shield documents were ultimately destroyed.

When the verdict came in against A. H. Robins in Connie Deemer's case, Tuttle was demoted and forced to give up all responsibility for handling Dalkon Shield matters. He claims he was fired by Forrest, then rehired after calling Zimmer and pleading for his job. Both Forrest and Zimmer deny that Tuttle was ever fired, but they don't deny he was demoted.

"That's a lie," Forrest recently said of Tuttle's contention that he was fired after losing Connie Deemer's case. "He wasn't fired, but I did relieve him of the responsibility for the Dalkon Shield. I told him—I was quite honest with him—that he certainly ought to recognize that his career position might be compromised but I wanted to give him another chance. I gave him another assignment in the law department and he stayed with Robins for a year thereafter, almost."

With the Connie Deemer case raising red flags in the company, and Forrest not satisfied with Tuttle's handling of the case, A. H. Robins turned to the prestigious Richmond law firm of McGuire, Woods and Battle. A. H. Robins had long and close ties with the firm; indeed, Zimmer had worked there before coming to A. H. Robins. The firm also represented Aetna Insurance, the company that provided products liability insurance for A. H. Robins and the Dalkon Shield.

Tuttle said he was careful not to discuss the destruction of documents with anyone inside of A. H. Robins, but he did feel a responsibility to tell the McGuire, Woods and Battle attorneys about it.

He said he told Alexander Slaughter and Rosewell Page, both attorneys with the Richmond firm, about the document destruction as part of their orientation process, sometime between March and June of 1975.

"I told Alex and Rosie that there had been a search," Tuttle said. "I told them who had done the searching, whose files had been searched, and that as a consequence there were considerable quantities of documents that had been burned."

Tuttle said he also told them what type of documents had been destroyed: "I described them as documents which appeared to me as the reviewer as legally damning where Robins' defense was concerned in respect of knowledge by top officers of the company and the lack of testing and the imperfect labeling." Slaughter and Page responded, Tuttle said, by asking how thorough the search had been.

During questioning by Sloan later in the deposition, Tuttle said the destruct order presented him with a dichotomy.

"A dichotomy between what?" Sloan asked.

"Between my duty to the client and a broader duty to the ladies that were or might become wearers of this device," Tuttle said.

Cudd called for a recess at 5 P.M., ending the first dramatic day of Tuttle's testimony. For the next three days, Tuttle would paint, scene by scene, a damning mural of what A. H. Robins looked like from the inside.

The theme of the mural was that of arrogant corporate executives repeatedly ignoring warnings from lower-level employees and blaming the Shield's problems on doctors, women—anybody but themselves. At the same time these executives were defending the Shield as a superior product and themselves as responsible businessmen, they were making sure their defense of the Shield would hold up by burning documents that indicated just the opposite was true.

Tuttle was careful but relaxed on the stand, a man who appeared glad to be unburdening himself of secrets he'd carried for nine-and-a-half years. He looked confident and at times seemed to be enjoying himself. At other times he seemed almost hurt by what had happened to him at A. H. Robins.

The documents Tuttle revealed during his first day of testimony became the focal point of the rest of the deposition. Some of these documents, however, were already known to plantiffs' attorneys. Other copies of the documents had escaped the 1975 search and destroy mission.

But there was one important memo in Tuttle's manila envelope that no one had seen before. It was referred to as Exhibit No. 10—Roy Smith's June 10, 1970, memo about copper in the Dalkon Shield. The memo was important because of the FDA's decision in 1972, based on information provided by A. H. Robins, that the Dalkon Shield did not contain enough copper to be classified as a drug. If the copper in the Shield leached from the device, then it would have been classified as a drug and subject to testing.

The Smith memo, written to C. E. Morton, a senior vice-president at A. H. Robins, with a carbon copy going to C. E. Bender, a vice-president, addressed the copper problem directly.

"The subject matter of the memo has to do with copper in the device and what the medical ramifications might be of that," Tuttle told the court.

"And in this memo," Ciresi said, "Mr. Smith states that according to his understanding, the inventors of the device observed that the device with copper was apparently lowering the pregnancy rate, correct?"

"That is what he states, yes sir," Tuttle agreed.

"And Mr. Smith states that he is troubled by the implication of that in the absence of full disclosure to the doctors," Ciresi said, "correct?"

Again, Tuttle agreed.

Ciresi sounded like he was reading from an old Perry Mason TV script, making incriminating statements and asking Tuttle to confirm them. Tuttle joined in, giving short, quick responses as if on cue.

"And A. H. Robins took the position in front of the FDA, both in '70 and in years subsequent to that, that the copper had no impact upon the effectiveness of it, correct?"

"Yes, sir," Tuttle said.

"And if the copper had had an effect on the pregnancy rate of the Dalkon Shield and Robins had so stated, that device would have been subject to FDA requirements for drugs that were in effect in 1970, correct?"

Sloan objected, breaking Ciresi's rhythm. He was promptly overruled.

"It would have been classified as a drug," Tuttle said, "and if it had been classified as a drug, it would have been subject to the new drug regulations."

"And that meant that it would have had to go through [FDA-required] testing, correct?" Ciresi said.

"Correct," Tuttle responded.

"And the Dalkon Shield wasn't subjected to any of that type of testing before marketing, was it, sir?" Ciresi asked.

"No, sir," Tuttle said.

In the memo, Smith wrote that he was concerned by what he termed A. H. Robins' implied warranty of the Shield. "If we sell the doctor a *device*," he wrote, underscoring the word device, "with no mention that the content of the material includes a copper salt which may contribute to the overall effectiveness, then it would seem clear that the doctor was buying a device and expecting the results to be attributable to that device."

"What troubles me," Smith continued in the memo, "is our implication to him, in the absence of full disclosure, that a device is doing the job whereas we would actually be selling a device to which we had added copper sulfate for the express purpose of getting an added drug effect."

Tuttle told the court that he had discussed the copper issue with Smith, Bender, Morton, and the doctors Owen, Clark, and Freund. Tuttle said he was "repeatedly assured by all concerned that copper ions either did not leach from the plastic or, if so, to such a minimal degree that there was no contraceptive effect."

Ciresi continued his questioning: "When you reviewed these documents, you found that that was false, though; is that correct, sir?"

"Consistent with other things I discovered," Tuttle said, "I found that I had not been told the truth."

Ciresi asked the critical question: "So Robins lied to the FDA, correct?"

"It would certainly appear so," Tuttle responded.

Ciresi turned his attention to another of the documents Tuttle had saved from destruction—Exhibit No. 14. It was a memo from Fred Clark to 10 different people in A. H. Robins, with additional copies also going to E. Claiborne Robins, Sr., Zimmer, and Thomas. The memo, dated August 24, 1970, was about an upcoming in-house meeting about the Shield.

The memo, Ciresi said, "refers to, among other things, the copper content of the Shield and the fact that there have been—or has been no testing with respect to its effect, both short- and long-term, in human beings, correct?"

"Yes, sir," Tuttle responded.

Tuttle said he believed that A. H. Robins also withheld from the custody of the FDA all memos mentioning the problem of the Shield's tail string wicking bacteria into the uterus.

"It was a cover-up, wasn't it?" Ciresi asked bluntly about A. H. Robins' dealing with the FDA in 1974 and 1975.

Tuttle, after objecting to the question himself and being overruled by

Cudd, answered: "Yes, sir."

Tuttle went on to recount a dramatic confrontation he had with Freund at a meeting in the medical department of A. H. Robins in the spring of 1975. At the time of the meeting, Tuttle said, the federal government was considering legislation or regulations that would hold corporate officials personally and criminally responsible for acts of their companies.

Tuttle was dismayed and frustrated at the company's handling of the Shield and, in a "fit of chagrin," turned to Freund in front of a group of A. H. Robins officials and said "words to the effect that Dr. Freund ought to be on his knees nightly praying to his God and mine . . . and thanking Him that he was not in that position where he would be subject to such a penalty because surely he would be doing hard time if the truth were ever known."

Tuttle reports that Freund "was outraged, stomped out of the meeting and never spoke to me again as long as I was with the Robins Company," Tuttle said. The other people at the meeting reacted with "stunned silence."

Freund, who retired from A. H. Robins at the end of 1977, recently described Tuttle as "peculiar." "He kept speaking in biblical sentences," Freund said. "Way back then Roger Tuttle would walk through the halls saying, 'We'll smite the Philistines.' I didn't know what he was talking about. He was peculiar and different then, and he is now."

A. H. Robins officials, of course, did not sit quietly by as Tuttle pulled damaging corporate memos from his manila envelope and made very damning statements about what went on inside the company.

John Taylor, vice-president of public affairs at A. H. Robins, issued a strong denial of Tuttle's testimony—a statement he'd read over the phone to Ciresi's secretary.

Ciresi pulled out a copy of the statement during the third, and final, day of the deposition and turned to Tuttle.

"Well, Mr. Taylor says that the allegations you've made are false," Ciresi said; then he read Taylor's statement to the court:

"The management of this company has never ordered nor permitted the destruction of Dalkon Shield documents and there is no reason to believe any such destruction ever occurred," the statement began. "Specifically, the company believes Mr. Tuttle's allegations to be absurd, without any foundation in fact, and the product of the imagination of a disgruntled former employee."

Almost a year later, at a May 1985 press conference, A. H. Robins accused Tuttle of falsifying a 1975 memo he claimed listed the initials of those company officials whose records were searched and of those who actually did the searching. Tuttle said he had written the memo during the weeks that the documents were destroyed; A. H. Robins claimed he wrote the memo two years later, after he had left the company. A. H. Robins also charged that, based on the expense account of another A. H. Robins employee, Tuttle was out of town during the time he said he was overseeing the document destruction.

When he completed Taylor's statement, Ciresi turned to Tuttle and said, "What's your response to that?"

"It doesn't surprise me, the fact that they would deny this," Tuttle said. "I would have assumed that they would have. And of course the fact that certain of the documents that were supposed to be destroyed have been preserved by me over the years would indicate that my allegations are true. And of course, with respect to my being a disgruntled former employee, that is a ridiculous statement. I left the Robins company to a better position financially and with greater responsibility, and then as a culmination of a desire of many years, subsequently left that position to teach. So I have nothing to gain or lose and have nothing to be disgruntled about."

Tuttle also revealed during the deposition that he had kept the many letters he had exchanged with Hugh Davis concerning the Shield. Tuttle said he kept the letters as "an insurance policy . . . to demonstrate that in fact I had been mislead, not only by Dr. Davis, but by the company itself in respect to what his real relationship was." Judge Cudd did not allow the letters into evidence because they were privileged communication between an attorney and his client.

On the final day of the deposition, Sloan picked up the questioning of Tuttle's honesty and motives for testifying.

"You were upset with Robins' medical department for not providing the information you felt you needed in the Deemer case," Sloan said.

"Frustrated would be a better word," Tuttle said.

"You were," Sloan said, "resentful of the fact that Forrest would not give you more legal support to handle the increasing load of Dalkon Shield litigation."

"Frustrated would be a better word," Tuttle said again, anticipating the direction Sloan was taking the questioning.

"And Forrest ignored your requests for help," Sloan asked.

"Well, he did not make a positive response," Tuttle said.

Sloan brought up several occasions in which Forrest had "chewed out" Tuttle for various misdeeds, such as going over Forrest's head to ask for more help in the legal department.

SLOAN: "And Mr. Forrest blamed you for the Deemer verdict?"

TUTTLE: "That is my impression, yes sir."

SLOAN: "And you felt that was grossly unfair?"

TUTTLE: "Well, I do feel it was unfair."

SLOAN: "And Mr. Forrest fired you at a time when you couldn't financially afford to lose your job."

TUTTLE: "That is correct."

"And you threatened to get even with the company?" Sloan asked, finally getting to the question that counted.

"Oh, no. No, sir," Tuttle said. "That is absolutely incorrect."

"You threatened to get even with Mr. Forrest," Sloan persisted.

"No, sir, that's not my province," Tuttle said. "It's in the hands of a higher being than you and I both."

Sloan came to his last question. "You're a born-again Christian, sir?"

"Yes, sir," Tuttle said.

With the deposition over, Tuttle seemed glad to have finally made public the guilt he carried within himself for so many years. Judge Miles Lord had inspired him to do it, and he felt better now that it was done. Perhaps Tuttle viewed his actions as an atonement for his earlier lack of courage.

There was also a bit of sadness in Tuttle. He still seemed to carry the pain of what he'd done, and let others do, a decade earlier.

"I'm not very smart, Mr. Ciresi," Tuttle said at one point in his testimony. "You know that by now. It's obvious as a result of this deposition and I guess that I was banged so much over a period of years about these things that I refused to believe what was obvious. I trusted the people that I was representing."

20

Sacrificial Wombs

"When I heard of all that [document destruction] . . . that's why I believe they should be paying all those women now. I can't stand a company that's not honest with their customers."
—Lillian Yin, director of the FDA's Office of Ob-Gyn Devices, April 1985.

In October 1984, a commercial with a most unusual message appeared nationally on network and cable television. A woman, in a soft, but serious tone, addressed viewers with the following 30-second message:

"This important health warning is for women still using the Dalkon Shield, an IUD birth control device obtained in the early to mid-1970s. There is substantial medical opinion that continued use of the Dalkon Shield may pose a serious personal health hazard and it should be removed. If you're still using the Dalkon Shield, its maker, A. H. Robins Company, will pay your doctor or clinic to remove it. It's that important."

Ten years after it was withdrawn from the market the Shield was finally being recalled. For the first time, A. H. Robins was telling women directly that they should go to their doctors and have their Shields removed.

The reason A. H. Robins decided to begin this $4.5 million recall campaign late in 1984 is not exactly clear. E. Claiborne Robins, Jr., in his official statement on the "removal program"—A. H. Robins does not like the term "recall"—said the company decided to do it "out of our concern for the health of these women, and quite frankly, our concern about the adverse publicity our company and the Dalkon Shield have received in recent months which we firmly believe is unwarranted. . . . Our company is committed to resolving this chapter in its history."

Certainly, adverse publicity during the nine months preceding the recall had taken its toll on the company. It had started with Judge Lord's speech in February 1984 and continued right through the summer with Roger Tuttle's testimony that A. H. Robins officials had destroyed documents. In late summer, "60 Minutes" reran its earlier segment on the Shield with an update. Later it broadcasted a second segment on Judge Lord.

Fletcher Owen, who spends 70 percent of his time testifying or otherwise speaking in A. H. Robins' defense, describes the first "60 Minutes" segment on the Shield as "a very negative discourse with women plaintiffs." Rather than evoking his empathy, the women presented in the segment seemed to have incited his scorn. "I thought they chose the most unattractive women to do that," Owen says of the women. "Some of them I thought were really wretched-looking people. It probably detracted from the message they were projecting—that is, bad, bad Robins."

With each new burst of news stories, hundreds more newly enlightened and angry women contacted attorneys. By the end of 1984, more than 12,000 women had sued or brought claims against the company; about 3,800 of those cases were still pending. In a recent study commissioned by A. H. Robins, the Washington, D.C., consulting firm Resource Planning Corporation estimated there will probably be another 8,300 suits filed by women before the Shield litigation finally concludes sometime after the year 2000.

But behind the scenes, other events may have also contributed to the recall. On September 19, 1984, Robert Manchester, a lawyer for the National Women's Health Network, wrote to the FDA about the recent deaths of three long-term Shield wearers. "These three deaths, if determined to be associated with the Dalkon Shield," wrote Manchester, "would clearly demonstrate that the Dalkon Shield risk is not over, even though the current number of wearers may be a small, residual population." Two of the deaths had occurred in Los Angeles, one in November 1981, the other in March 1984. The third woman had died in New Orleans in April 1983.

The FDA began an investigation of the deaths.

Also, new information about A. H. Robins' "Cadillac of IUD studies," the Ten Investigator Prospective Study, was about to come to light, information that might make the study look more like an Edsel than a Cadillac.

The new information concerned one of the 10 studies that, collectively, made up what was known as the Ten Investigator Prospective Study. It had been conducted at Thad Earl's old clinic in Defiance, Ohio, although after Earl had moved to Arizona. Of the 149 women who had been inserted with a Shield in the study, only one was reported to have developed PID later. This gave the study a PID rate of .7 percent, one of the lowest among the 10 studies. All 10 studies combined reported a PID rate of 3.0 percent.

Early in 1984, Minnesota attorney Patricia Hartmann called the Defiance clinic and persuaded a doctor there to review the 120 medical records from the study that could still be found. The doctor, Robert Barnett, was astonished at what he discovered. Instead of one pelvic infection, he found 18 definite pelvic infections, and possibly as many as 31. This meant the Defiance study had a PID rate of at least 12.1 percent. It could have actually been higher, for there were 13 questionable infections and 29 missing records.

Barnett wrote to A. H. Robins on July 13, 1984, telling the company that his review of the records showed a PID rate 15 to 20 times higher than A. H. Robins had originally reported from the study. But it was not until January 1985, six months later, that Fletcher Owen told Barnett that A. H. Robins would be reviewing the data from the study.

In late March 1985, A. H. Robins officials acknowledged to Thomas Morris, a reporter from the *Richmond Times-Dispatch*, that there might be some inaccuracies in the Defiance study. Some of the data sheets from the study, the company acknowledged, were left blank next to the question of whether PID was present in the patient. "Looking through [with] 20-20 hindsight," Fletcher Owen told Morris, "I'd go as far as to say that a data sheet that didn't have a PID box checked yes or no, in my opinion, should have been returned to the investigator." (The data sheets were forms that were supposed to be filled out by doctors while examining the women in the study. The forms were later sent to A. H. Robins where the doctor's comments were interpreted before being entered into a computer.)

The data sheets from the Defiance study are not the only ones to raise questions about the accuracy of the Ten Investigator Prospective Study. According to attorneys who have looked at the sheets from the 10 studies, some of the sheets have "do not quote" and "do not count" written on them next to such symptoms as abnormal bleeding, vaginal odor, or hysterectomy—the kinds of symptoms that strongly suggest the presence of PID. Whether or not these instructions were followed, their presence certainly raises the question of whether or not all incidents of PID were noted for the final statistical analysis.

Something else happened in the fall of 1984 that may have persuaded A. H. Robins to issue a recall of the Shield. The Minneapolis law firm of Robins, Zelle, Larson and Kaplan negotiated the settlement of 198 Shield lawsuits for a reported $38 million—a record for Shield settlements. The individual settlements ranged from $5,000 to $3 million, with the average being about $192,000.

Michael Ciresi of Robins-Zelle says that his law firm pushed for a recall during the settlement process. He says he told A. H. Robins attorneys that, unless there was some strong action to get the Shield out of women, Robins-Zelle planned to take the plaintiffs' cases directly to the company's full board of directors. Ciresi says his firm had decided to make a videotape using excerpts from the testimony of A. H. Robins' top officials to show the board members how they had been misled about the Shield and to argue for a recall.

A. H. Robins decided to initiate the recall before Robins-Zelle could make its presentation, says Ciresi. A. H. Robins officials, however, contend Robins-Zelle had nothing to do with the recall. Fletcher Owen said the recall was done for "a composite of medical reasons and legal reasons, and certainly I have to give the lion's share to the latter." It was done to silence the critics "who said we hadn't gone far enough" in warning women about the Shield, he said, and "out of concern for those women who continue to use it. We decided that this thing should be carried down to the level of the user and that hopefully that would put this matter to rest. We're tired of this. We've had almost . . . 15 years of the Dalkon Shield."

Former U.S. Attorney General Griffin Bell, who had represented A. H. Robins in its suit against Judge Lord, said in May 1985 that it was he who urged A. H. Robins to conduct the recall campaign. "We needed this as an act of good faith to warn people about continued wearing of the Dalkon Shield," Bell said.

Whatever the reasons behind A. H. Robins' recall, company executives from E. Claiborne Robins, Jr., on down were—and are—insisting that the Shield is still a good product, no worse and perhaps better in design than other IUDs still on the market. The Shield has simply been the victim of a biased press and greedy plaintiffs' attorneys, former A. H. Robins President William Zimmer and other A. H. Robins officials said recently. From their viewpoint, it seems that everybody—from Howard Tatum to Roger Tuttle—has some reason to do A. H. Robins harm.

But with the recall, A. H. Robins finally did what its critics had urged it to do years earlier: it told women directly to have their Shields removed.

Immediately after the recall was announced the company was receiving up to 1,500 calls a day from women concerned about the Shield. As of mid-April 1985, A. H. Robins had received more than 18,000 calls (including some from "kooks," according to A. H. Robins attorney William Forrest) and had removed more than 3,200 Shields from women.

But the thousands of calls did not account for all of the women who might be wearing the Shield. Of the 4.5 million Shields manufactured by A. H. Robins, about 1.7 million of the devices were shipped overseas, most often to poor, developing countries. Advertisements announcing A. H. Robins' recall appeared in Australia and Great Britain; but not in El Salvador, Uganda, Morocco, or most of the other countries (approximately 80) where the Shield was routinely inserted in women during the first half of the 1970s.

One of A. H. Robins' largest customers for its overseas sales was the U.S. Agency for International Development (AID), which purchased and shipped nearly 700,000 Shields to about 70 developing countries. When A. H. Robins recalled the Shield in October 1984, AID officials began a review of their past efforts to have the device removed from women around the world. Ironically, it was Russel Thomsen, one of the earliest and strongest critics of A. H. Robins, who was in charge of conducting this review.

Thomsen had been out of the Shield controversy for many years. After testifying about the dangers of the Shield at the 1973 Fountain Hearings and at Connie Deemer's trial in 1975, Thomsen decided not to become a "professional witness" and returned to practicing medicine for the Army, where he was eventually promoted to the rank of colonel. His involvement with the Shield, however, had sparked his interest in world population problems in general and IUDs in particular. In addition to gathering one of the world's largest collection of IUDs and writing an atlas of IUDs, Thompsen went to work in AID's office of population. He also continued to practice medicine at the DeWitt Army Hospital at Fort Belvoir in Northern Virginia.

According to Thomsen's report on overseas sales of the Shield, published in February 1985, AID's interest and use of IUDs had begun early in the 1960s with the development of the new plastic IUDs. By the end of that decade the agency had distributed millions of IUDs overseas, primarily the Lippes Loop. "It was," Thomsen wrote of the Loop in his report, "a known, tested entity. Furthermore, clinicians were trained in both the Loop's insertion technique and [in how] to deal with its potential complications." Indeed, Thomsen noted, AID was so familiar and comfortable with the Loop that it turned down a request to use the Majzlin Spring overseas, presumably before the dangers of the Spring were fully known.

Similar requests about the Shield, however, were not turned down. "A.I.D.'s use of the Dalkon Shield followed pressure exerted by both requests from the field [AID's overseas offices] and marketing contacts by personnel from A. H. Robins," Thomsen said. The first request from an AID field office for a Shield came on June 17, 1970, when the AID Mission in Morocco sent a cable asking if it could purchase 25,000 Shields from the Dalkon Corporation. (This was five days after the Shield had been sold to A. H. Robins, but presumably that news had not yet reached Morocco.) The request was eventually approved and nine months later 1,920 Shields were sent to Morocco.

By September 1970, it was no longer the Dalkon Corporation, but A. H. Robins, that was directing the Shield's sales effort, and the approach to AID was more aggressive. On September 15, 1970, Robert Nickless, the international marketing manager for A. H. Robins, sent 32 Shields to Dr. R. T. Ravenholt, director of AID's office of population. "This intrauterine device does look promising," Ravenholt wrote to Nickless. "We will immediately send three of the cartons [of Shields] to Pakistan and send the balance to one or more countries where they might be put to best use."

The door to the overseas market really opened for A. H. Robins when Dr. Gladys Dodds, the medical director of the Family Planning Association of Hong Kong, asked for a large number of Shields. The Dalkon Corporation had earlier sent her a few sample Shields, and she wanted more. In November 1970, AID arranged for A. H. Robins to send 960 multiparous Shields to Dodds. The company provided the Shields free of charge. Apparently satisfied with the Shields, Dodds and the International Planned Parenthood Federation asked AID to provide funding for as many as 20,000 Shields three months later. On April 21, 1971, the General Services Administration, at the behest of AID, shipped the first of 10,176 Dalkon Shields to Dodds.

"From that purchase, the Dalkon Shield assumed an ever increasing importance in A.I.D.'s IUD program until the last shipment was made by [the General Services Administration] on 15 April 1974," Thomsen wrote in his report. "Especially close was the working relationship developed by Robert W. Nickless, Director of International Marketing for A. H. Robins, with A.I.D."

Thomsen, who had been publicly attacking the Shield during the time AID had been shipping it overseas in the early 1970s, now found himself, 10 years later, trying to justify AID's actions in his 1985 report. "The implication that A.I.D.'s acceptance and utilization of the Dalkon Shield was both immediate and major must be tempered by historical perspective," Thomsen wrote. "It needs to be recalled that at that time the FDA did not regulate IUDs, in fact, did not officially know which IUDs were on the market. Individual physicians, major agencies such as A.I.D., and family planning organizations had no regulatory guidance on devices. In that millieu [sic], reliance was placed on major pharmaceutical firms, such as A. H. Robins, that claims for the pharmaceuticals they were marketing were, in fact, backed up by reputable and reproducible evidence."

In 1971 AID sent 20,064 Shields to Hong Kong and Uganda. Shipments picked up sharply in 1972 and by mid-1974 the Agency had shipped almost 700,000 Shields to about 70 countries around the world.

When A. H. Robins suspended marketing of the Shield in June 1974, AID sent out a message to its field offices warning of the link between septic abortion and the Shield and recommended that use of the device be discontinued. When the FDA held a press conference in early July 1974 advising physicians not to insert any more Shields in their patients, AID sent a similar message to its field offices.

On February 28, 1975, about a month after A. H. Robins issued a notice telling its detailmen to begin collecting and returning unused Shields, AID issued a cable to its field offices "giving instructions for the return of unused stocks of Dalkon Shields for reimbursement by A. H. Robins," Thomsen said. "No recommendation that Dalkon Shields should be removed from women successfully using them for contraception had been made by A.I.D. to this point, this being in line with FDA and manufacturer pronouncements on the subject." By January 25, 1976, Thomsen said in his report, "all known A.I.D.-furnished stocks of Dalkon shields were returned to A. H. Robins or destroyed as instructed by the company. A total of 328,997 Dalkon shields was returned to A. H. Robins for which payment of $196,775 was reimbursed to A.I.D."

The agency was apparently satisfied that it had taken care of the Shield problem. But then in September 1980, A. H. Robins issued its "Dear Doctor Number 2" letter recommending to doctors that the Shield be removed from all women. In late November, AID cabled its field offices to pass on the A. H. Robins recommendation. It also asked AID officials in various countries to meet with local population officials to develop plans to notify women about having the Shield removed. "Cable responses from field population officers indicated wide dissemination of this warning message," Thomsen said in his report, "and that in response to this and previous action [by AID] there appeared to be few women still using Dalkon Shields."

Yet another AID cable went out in 1983 after the Centers for Disease Control found that women using the Shield ran a risk of getting PID five times greater than women using other IUDs. "Again, this cable stated that any remaining Dalkon Shields should be removed," Thomsen wrote, "and that this information should be shared with host country counterparts."

As part of its October 1984 recall campaign, Thomsen noted, A. H. Robins "notified the Ambassadors to the United States of the 79 countries in which Dalkon Shields were distributed of this 'recall' effort and asked the Ambassadors' counsel as to whether a Dalkon Shield information program would be appropriate in their countries."

Thomsen said AID monitored the recall closely and concluded that a minimum of 47 percent—or 328,997—of the Shields sent out by AID had been accounted for. That, of course, left 53 percent—or 368,295—of the Shields unaccounted for. In his report for AID, however, Thomsen downplays the possibility that the Shields are still in use. "The thorough response which A.I.D. got to its world-wide cables on the Dalkon Shield indicates that few Dalkon Shields are likely still in use," Thomsen concluded.

But reports from officials in several countries, as well as American attorneys concerned about overseas sales, indicate there may be many women still wearing the Shield.

"There were . . . around 100,000 [Shields] or better sold in Australia," Boston attorney Robert Manchester said. "The problem is that it is impossible to verify how many devices were in fact inserted in Australia."

Manchester's concern was echoed by Martina Langley, an Austin, Texas, attorney who has spent several years working with the poor in clinics in El Salvador. Langley said she saw Shields being inserted in women as late as 1980 in El Salvador; and that the doctors there and in other Central American countries have shown very little concern about women who still wear the Shield. Thomsen's conclusion that few women are still wearing the device "is a hypocritical joke," Langley said.

Record-keeping in El Salvador's medical clinics is atrocious, if it exists at all, Langley continued, so there is no way to know how many Shields were inserted or how many have been removed. And even worse, she said, neither A. H. Robins nor AID has conducted a publicity campaign to let women know that they should have the Shield removed. "Both AID and Robins have a duty to make sure that all the IUDs were destroyed or returned, and not just take anybody's word for it," Langley said. "Robins has a plant right in San Salvador and if they would give five cents apiece for [Shields], they would have gotten every one of them."

Inexpensive radio campaigns would probably be adequate to get the word out to most women in developing countries, Langley said, but her requests to A. H. Robins to run such a campaign have gone unanswered.

In April 1985, after Langley went public with her concerns, AID announced a new series of studies to be conducted in conjunction with the Centers for Disease Control to try to determine if women in foreign countries are still wearing the Shield. The studies were to concentrate on El Salvador, Costa Rica, Kenya, and Tanzania—four countries where large numbers of the Shield were used.

Thomsen, however, said he stands by the conclusions of his report that AID's efforts to remove the Shield from women in developing countries were successful. "We have data from a lot of sources to back that up," he said. But the new studies, to be completed in late 1985, should show if the AID recall was as thorough as Thomsen believes it was.

Langley is pleased that the studies are going to be conducted, but remains critical of A. H. Robins' failure to conduct publicity campaigns to directly inform women in developing countries about the dangers of the Shield.

"I'm not trying to do them in," she said of A. H. Robins. "I just want to get it [the Shield] out of the women."

20

Epilogue

"If you took all these women [who have been injured by the Dalkon Shield] and put them in a stadium, then you'd see the real tragedy of this story."
— Ken Green, plaintiffs' attorney.

On May 3, 1985, more than a decade after a jury in Wichita, Kansas, in the first ruling against A. H. Robins, awarded Connie Deemer $85,000 for injuries she suffered from wearing the Shield, another Wichita jury handed down another devastating verdict against the pharmaceutical company. Bradley Post, who won that first case against A. H. Robins, was once again the plaintiffs attorney. This time he was representing Loretta Tetuan, a 33-year-old woman who had undergone a hysterectomy in 1979 as a result of a PID infection that she claimed was caused by the Shield.

The jury awarded her the largest judgment in the 10 years of the Shield litigation—$8.9 million—$1.4 million in actual damages and $7.5 million in punitive damages. A. H. Robins spokesman Roscoe Puckett immediately said the company would appeal the judgment and then repeated a statement the company has been using, with decreasing effectiveness, for 10 years: "The company does not believe the Dalkon Shield caused the plaintiffs injuries."

A month before the conclusion of Loretta Tetuan's trial, two major federally sponsored studies appeared, linking use of IUDs directly to infertility for the first time. The studies, sponsored by the National Institute of Child Health and Human Development, found that women

236

who have not had children were twice as likely to become infertile if they used an IUD. The risk increased according to the type of IUD a woman wore, with the Shield ranked as the device presenting the greatest risk of infertility. A woman who wore a Shield faced a three to seven times greater risk of being sterile than a woman who hadn't worn a Shield, the reports said.

Yet A. H. Robins officials, from E. Claiborne Robins, Jr., on down, continue to deny that the Shield is less safe or less effective than any other IUD. For A. H. Robins attorney William Forrest, this denial appears to extend into his personal life as well. In a deposition taken in February 1984, Forrest said his wife had a hysterectomy shortly after her own Shield had been removed in 1975. But he recalled surprisingly few specifics surrounding the operation.

"Did her doctor advise her that her hysterectomy was in any way related to the Dalkon Shield?" asked Robins-Zelle attorney Mike Ciresi during the deposition.

"Not that I know of, no, sir," responded Forrest.

"Did you ever ask her that?"

"Pardon?"

"Did you ever ask her that?"

"I don't recall," Forrest said. "I may have asked her that. I don't recall the doctor telling her that."

"You just don't know one way or the other?"

"Pardon?"

"You just don't know one way or the other as you sit here today?" Ciresi repeated.

"That's correct, sir."

Forrest and most of the other A. H. Robins officials who played key roles in the Shield story remain with the company today. Some, like Forrest, Ken Moore, and Roy Smith, were promoted to vice-presidencies within the company. William Zimmer has retired from the presidency but remains active in Shield matters for A. H. Robins. E. Claiborne Robins, Sr., although reportedly in poor health, remains chairman of the board, the patriarch of the company that his father founded and the one his son is trying to save from financial disaster.

A. H. Robins had, as of April 1985, already paid $260 million to settle 7,700 Shield claims and could spend as much as $1 billion before Shield litigation is expected to end, sometime early in the next century. It has set aside a $615 million reserve fund to cover the anticipated legal claims, but company officials say that the fund may not be enough to cover punitive as well as compensatory damages arising out of the claims. Also it may not cover lawsuits filed overseas.

A. H. Robins reported that financial losses in 1984 as a result of the Shield were staggering. The company reported a net loss of $461.6 million for the year, a sum larger than the net worth of the entire company. It was also a loss large enough to wipe out all shareholder dividends for the next two years.

In response to a lawsuit filed several years ago by some shareholders, the company also agreed, without admitting any guilt, to set up a $6.9 million fund to reimburse shareholders who bought stock in the company between 1971 and 1974, the period during which the Shield was marketed by A. H. Robins.

Late in 1984, A. H. Robins announced that it had settled yet another lawsuit—with its insurer, Aetna Casualty and Surety Company. Aetna and A. H. Robins were involved in a four-year lawsuit about how much the insurance company should be required to pay in Shield cases. The lawsuit was settled when Aetna agreed to add $70 million to its coverage of the Shield, bringing the total amount of insurance money available from Aetna for Shield litigation to $369 million.

A. H. Robins blames many people for the fall of the Shield and the company's resultant financial woes—women, doctors, lawyers, journalists, judges, and others who it believes have hidden reasons for wanting the Shield portrayed as a dangerous device. A company under siege, it is behaving with a siege mentality. Executives, both former and current, exhibit a strong "us against them" attitude.

One of the company's major antagonists, the Minnesota law firm of Robins, Zelle, Larson and Kaplan, is no longer representing Shield victims. The firm dropped out of Shield litigation during the fall of 1984 after its $38 million settlement of 198 cases with A. H. Robins. Although Robins-Zelle attorneys say their dropping out of the litigation was not part of the settlement with A. H. Robins, critics of the firm accuse it of selling out. Robins-Zelle attorneys, however, point out that they have made all the evidence and documents gathered by the firm available to attorneys all over the country, charging only a minimum fee to cover duplicating costs of documents. Indeed, Robins-Zelle has published a free catalogue of Shield materials from which attorneys can place orders for documents and other items they might need in their lawsuits against A. H. Robins.

Today, Michael Ciresi heads a team of Robins-Zelle attorneys representing the government of India in claims arising out of the 1984 Bhopal tragedy in India, where more than 2,000 people were killed and about 200,000 injured as a result of a leak of methyl isocyanate at a plant owned by a subsidiary of the Union Carbide Corporation.

On May 19, 1985, Judge Miles Lord, whose rulings played a major role in Robins-Zelle's success with the Shield litigation, announced he was stepping down from the federal bench. Lord, 65, said he wanted to "smell the roses" and devote more time to his family. His dramatic speech to the A. H. Robins executives had not been the final controversial act of his very controversial career. Late in 1984, Lord again drew national attention to his courtroom when he gave probation rather than lengthy prison terms to two peace activists who had smashed computer equipment at the Sperry Corporation plant near Minneapolis. He used the sentencing of the two as a platform to attack Sperry's overcharging the federal government for defense contracts and to criticize the nation's glamorization of weapons.

Lord was one of the few true champions of the women who were injured by the Shield. It was a role that should have been performed years earlier by the FDA. But the agency, unlike Lord, was not able to overcome its bureaucratic timidity and step forward to protect the rights of women aggressively.

FDA officials have consistently blamed their ineffectiveness in the Shield tragedy on the lack of a strong law giving them the power to act. That law, the 1976 Medical Device Amendments to the Food, Drug, and Cosmetic Act, is now on the books, but questions have been raised about its effectiveness. In a 1983 review of the way the law was being used to protect the public from devices such as the Shield, the General Accounting Office found that the "FDA did not have a comprehensive system to collect and analyze data on medical device problems and their causes and severity."

The report also makes the disturbing observation that "device manufacturers and distributors are not required to notify the FDA when they become aware of a death, injury, or hazard caused by a medical device." The FDA is still trusting companies to voluntarily acknowledge problems with their products that harm those who use them.

It is just such a trusting relationship between the FDA and the medical and pharmaceutical communities that allowed the Shield to be inserted in millions of women throughout the world.

Pam Van Duyn filed a lawsuit against the A. H. Robins Company in 1979. She won the case five years later, in March 1984, when a Eugene, Oregon, jury awarded her $147,500 in compensatory damages. A. H. Robins attorneys, however, immediately appealed the award, and almost a year later, Pam had yet to receive any of the money.

As far as Pam is concerned, however, no amount of money can

replace the emotional and physical agony she has gone through. Because of her Shield-related medical problems, Pam says, she began to feel unattractive and worthless as a woman. She also felt her husband would be better off with someone who could give him children. "I saw my husband playing with his nieces," Pam says, "and I thought 'he is not infertile, I am.' " In 1980, she and her husband separated briefly. "She felt she was just this neutered object walking the face of the globe," Pam's husband, Jim, says of that difficult period in their lives. Their marriage now seems solid. "I just love her a lot," says Jim. "It's our love for each other that helped us prevail."

In 1983, Pam had an operation to remove her left Fallopian tube and ovary, which had repeatedly and painfully flared up from the chronic infection caused by the Shield. Then in January 1984, Pam underwent yet another operation, this one involving delicate microsurgery to clear the scar tissue from her right Fallopian tube. It was her one remaining hope of having children. But several months after the operation, Pam had yet to become pregnant. The damage to her Fallopian tube may have been too extensive to repair.

Linda Towle was more fortunate. The microsurgery done on her Fallopian tubes worked and on July 8, 1981, she gave birth by Cesarean section to a healthy son, whom she and her husband named Joshua. To have another child, however, Linda would have to undergo more microsurgery, for the scarring has returned to block her Fallopian tubes again. Linda does not feel she can go through the trauma of yet another operation. Linda has also sued A. H. Robins, although her case has not yet gone to trial.

Peggy and Melissa Mample's case did go to trial, with a jury eventually awarding more than $1.4 million for Melissa's injuries. The money has been put into a trust fund for Melissa to draw upon during the rest of her life. Peggy has two sons, Shuyler and Shane, both born without physical handicaps. She has recently remarried and has started her own cabinet-building business in Boise. Melissa is doing well in school and is active in the Special Olympics. Peggy hopes that one day her daughter will be able to lead an independent life, despite her handicaps.

Cynthia Parker today lives with her husband and four children in a suburb of Minneapolis, in the same house she and her husband had picked out after she became pregnant while wearing the Shield. Cynthia sued A. H. Robins, eventually settling out of court. She had decided against going to trial after following Brenda S.'s trial in the Minneapolis newspapers. "I didn't want to go through that," she says. "I didn't think I was strong enough."

Cynthia, like other Shield victims, cannot forget what the device did to her. "Something was done to me that should have been illegal," she says. "It killed my baby and it almost killed me."

When asked recently what he would say to these and other women who have suffered because they wore the Shield, former A. H. Robins President William Zimmer stood up abruptly from his chair in a small conference room at A. H. Robins' Richmond headquarters.

"Ah, hell, don't ask me a question like that," he said angrily. "This is absurd. Anyone who has suffered for any reason you're going to have great compassion for. Now I'm convinced that the Dalkon Shield is no different than other IUDs." The true victim in the Shield story, he insists, is A. H. Robins.

"We're not only being victimized by the plaintiff's bar, but we've been victimized by the press . . . I feel strongly about this . . . and these women, of course, who have suffered, it's a sad thing and I've great compassion for them. [But with] a lot of them it's not attributable to the Dalkon Shield . . . it could have happened with any other IUD."

He then walked out of the room.

But Pam Van Duyn can't walk away from the despair she sometimes feels because she cannot have children. Linda Towle can't walk away from the memory of years of physical and emotional pain as she underwent eight operations before finally succeeding in having a baby. Peggy Mample can't walk away from her handicapped child; indeed, her daughter, Melissa, can't walk at all. And Cynthia Parker can't walk away from her memories of a daughter born dead.

For these women, and thousands of others like them around the world, the story of the Shield is a very real and lasting nightmare of pain and sadness.

Time Line

1962

April 30–May 1, 1962: First International Conference on Intrauterine Contraception convenes in New York City.

1963

A. H. Robins' annual sales top $50 million for the first time. The company makes its first public offering of stock.

1964

Hugh Davis and Edmund Jones begin work on the INCON. Davis opens a family planning clinic at Johns Hopkins Hospital.

Irwin Lerner forms Lerner Laboratories.

1965

A. H. Robins stock is listed on the New York Stock Exchange.

1967

December 1967: Davis and Lerner discuss IUDs.

1968

January–August 1968: Lerner works on the design for the Dalkon Shield.

March 19, 1968: The FDA considers classifying all IUDs as drugs rather than devices.

September 1968: Davis begins his 12-month 640-patient study of the Dalkon Shield using only a one-sized model of the device.

November 1968: Lerner applies for a patent for the Dalkon Shield.

1969

January 1969: Davis, Lerner, and Robert Cohn form the Dalkon Corporation.

September 1969: Davis ends his 12-month study of the Shield.

October 1969: Davis submits a paper on his study to the *American Journal of Obstetrics & Gynecology.*

October 1969–June 1970: Davis and Lerner add copper to the Shield and make other design changes. Sales of the Shield by the Dalkon Corporation begin.

December 1969: Nulliparous, or small, model of the Shield is designed. Dr. Thad Earl visits Davis in Baltimore and Lerner in Connecticut.

1970

January 14, 1970: Senator Gaylord Nelson, chairman of the Sub-Committee on Monopoly of the Select Committee of Small Business begins hearings on the dangers of the Pill. Davis is the lead-off witness.

February 1970: Davis' article on his 12-month Shield study is published in the *American Journal of Obstetrics & Gynecology.*

April 4, 1970: Earl buys a 7.5 interest in the Dalkon Corporation.

May 1970: John McClure, a salesman for A. H. Robins, meets Earl at a medical exhibition in Bedford Springs, Pennsylvania.

May 28, 1970: Roy Smith, Dr. Edward Davis, and Dr. Fred Clark fly to Defiance, Ohio, to evaluate the Dalkon Shield at Earl's medical office.

June 8, 1970: Oscar Klioze talks to Lerner about the Shield and discovers that no formal stability or accelerated aging tests have been conducted on the Shield. Also, Fred Clark visits Davis in Baltimore and learns that the raw data from Davis' study shows a higher pregnancy rate for the Shield than Davis reported in the *American Journal of Obstetrics & Gynecology.*

June 9, 1970: Fred Clark writes a memo (the so-called secret memo) about his June 8 meeting with Davis.

June 10, 1970: Roy Smith writes a memo to C. E. Morton, A. H. Robins general manager, expressing his concern about selling the Shield to doctors without fully disclosing that copper sulfate had been added to the device to enhance its contraceptive effectiveness.

June 11, 1970: Dr. Jack Freund notes in a memo that Davis' one-year follow-up period for his study is not long enough to project pregnancy figures with any confidence.

June 12, 1970: A. H. Robins purchases the Dalkon Shield from the Dalkon Corporation for $750,000 plus a 10 percent royalty.

June 1970: Lerner warns Bob Nickless that the Dalkon Shield's tail string has a "wicking tendency."

October–November 1970: A. H. Robins makes design changes in the Dalkon Shield.

December 1970: A. H. Robins begins its two-year Ten Investigator Prospective Study of the Shield.

1971

January 1971: A. H. Robins begins its national marketing campaign for the Dalkon Shield.

April 1971: A. H. Robins officials meet with the FDA and argue that the Shield should be classified as a device rather than a drug. The officials claim copper was added to the Shield to improve its radiopacity rather than its effectiveness as a contraceptive.

June 1971: Wayne Crowder conducts experiments on the Shield's tail string and concludes that it wicks.

September 1971: Earl publishes his favorable article on the Shield in *American Family Physician*. Davis publishes his book, *The Intrauterine Device for Contraception*.

October 1971: A. H. Robins hires Wilcox and Williams to promote the Shield directly to women.

1972

February 1972: Ken Moore acknowledges in a memo that the Shield's nylon string may deteriorate during use. Also, Lester Preston writes a memo criticizing the work of Dr. Donald Ostergard, one of the investigators for A. H. Robins' Ten Investigator Prospective Study.

May–June 1972: National sales of the Shield begin to decline.

May 4, 1972: The FDA sends a letter to A. H. Robins stating that upon review of the data supplied by the company, the Shield will be classified as a device rather than a drug.

June 23, 1972: Earl writes a letter to John Burke of A. H. Robins warning about septic abortion and other problems with the Shield.

November 1972: A. H. Robins begins a second advertising blitz for the Shield with an eight-page "Progress Report" advertisement.

1973

February 28, 1973: The FDA issues a regulation that IUDs with active ingredients will be classified as drugs rather than devices.

March 22, 1973: Legislation is introduced in Congress to give FDA authority to regulate medical devices.

March 30, 1973: A 31-year-old Arizona woman dies as the result of a spontaneous septic abortion. She had been wearing a Dalkon Shield when she became pregnant.

May 25, 1973: The FDA seizes 9,000 Majzlin Spring IUDs.

May 31, 1973: Dr. Russel Thomsen testifies at the House Intergovernmental Relations Subcommittee's hearings on the regulation of medical devices.

June 1973: Both the FDA and A. H. Robins learn of the septic abortion death of the Arizona woman.

November 1973: A. H. Robins officials have conversations with Dr. Donald Christian about septic abortion deaths.

December 1973: A. H. Robins learns that Christian is about to publish an article about the Dalkon Shield and septic abortion.

1974

January 1974: A study from the Kaiser-Permanente Medical Center in Sacramento, California, reports a 5.6 percent pregnancy rate and a 28.7 percent removal rate for the Dalkon Shield.

February 15, 1974: A. H. Robins' Septic Abortion Conference is held in Richmond. Dr. Howard Tatum leaves the conference to begin studies on the Shield's tail string.

March 1974: A study conducted at the Beth Israel Hospital in Boston reports a 10.1 percent pregnancy rate for the Dalkon Shield.

May 8, 1974: A. H. Robins sends a "Dear Doctor" letter to 120,000 physicians advising them to take special precautions if a patient becomes pregnant while wearing the Shield.

May 24, 1974: In an internal progress report for the Dalkon Shield, Roger Tuttle is quoted as being opposed to removing the Shield from the market because such an action would be a "confession of liability."

May 28, 1974: The Planned Parenthood Federation instructs its 183 clinics to stop prescribing the Dalkon Shield immediately because of the threat of septic abortion.

June 1974: Christian's article on the connection between the Shield and fatal cases of sepsis appears in the *American Journal of Obstetrics & Gynecology.*

June 11, 1974: Dr. Fred Clark appears before an FDA Ob-Gyn Device Panel to defend the Shield.

June 26, 1974: FDA Commissioner Alexander Schmidt requests that A. H. Robins suspend marketing the Dalkon Shield until its "questionable safety" can be reviewed.

June 28, 1974: A. H. Robins suspends marketing the Dalkon Shield.

July 1974: The Centers for Disease Control report that its survey of 34,544 physicians revealed that fatal septic abortions occurred twice as frequently among Shield users as among women who wore other IUDs.

July 30, 1974: The FDA sends A. H. Robins a written request for information regarding the Dalkon Shield's safety and efficacy.

August 15, 1974: A. H. Robins President William Zimmer asks 15 A. H. Robins employees to search their files for any written communications regarding the Shield's tail string.

August 21–22, 1974: The FDA's Ad Hoc Committee holds hearings on the Dalkon Shield. Howard Tatum reports on the Shield's tail string and its wicking tendency.

August 1974: The FDA confirms that 11 women have died and another 209 have become seriously ill from septic abortions while wearing the Dalkon Shield.

October 30, 1974: The FDA's Ad Hoc Committee issues a final report that calls for a continuation of the moratorium on the marketing of the Dalkon Shield.

December 20, 1974: FDA Commissioner Alexander Schmidt announces that sales of the Shield will resume under a formal registry and reporting system.

1975

February 8, 1975: A Wichita jury awards Connie Deemer $10,000 in compensatory damages and $75,000 in punitive damages for medical injuries she sustained as a result of using the Dalkon Shield.

Mid–1975: A. H. Robins hires the law firm of McGuire, Woods, and Battle to handle its Shield litigation.

August 8, 1975: A. H. Robins abandons plans to remarket the Shield, but continues to claim the device is safe and effective.

August 15, 1975: The final results of A. H. Robins' two-year Ten Investigator Prospective Study are compiled, but not made public.

1976

The first multi-district litigation (MDL) discovery process is completed. By mid-year, 533 Dalkon Shield suits demanding $480 million in punitive and compensatory damages are pending before courts throughout the country.

May 28, 1976: The Medical Device Amendments are enacted as part of the Food, Drug, and Cosmetic Act. The amendments require a company to demonstrate the safety and efficacy of an IUD before it is marketed.

1977

May 10, 1977: The FDA publishes a regulation requiring uniform physician and patient labeling for all IUDs.

December 8, 1977: Attorneys Aaron Levine and Bradley Post make a statement to the FDA's Obstetrics and Gynecological Medical Devices Panel in which they ask the panel and the FDA to tell women still wearing the Shield to have it removed immediately.

Attorneys from McGuire, Woods, and Battle begin to commission studies on the Dalkon Shield. These later became known as the "secret studies" because the results were not made public.

1980

September 25, 1980: A. H. Robins issues a second "Dear Doctor" letter to 200,000 physicians recommending that the Shield be removed from women still wearing it.

1981

November 1981: A woman in Los Angeles dies, allegedly as a result of a Dalkon Shield-related infection.

1982

June 6, 1982: A Minnesota jury awards Brenda S. $1.75 million for her Dalkon Shield injuries.

The MDL discovery process is reopened briefly to allow for the collection of more documents.

1983

April 1983: A woman in New Orleans dies, allegedly as a result of wearing a Dalkon Shield.

1984

February 8, 1984: Judge Miles Lord issues an order for A. H. Robins to produce thousands of new Dalkon Shield documents.

February 29, 1984: Judge Lord makes his speech to three A. H. Robins executives in which he asks them to stop the "monstrous mischief" of their company and recall the Dalkon Shield.

March 1984: A Los Angeles woman dies, allegedly as a result of wearing a Dalkon Shield.

April 1984: A. H. Robins files two complaints against Judge Lord, claiming he had "grossly abused his office" by lecturing three A. H. Robins executives.

July 13, 1984: Dr. Robert Barnett of Defiance, Ohio, writes to A. H. Robins officials to tell them that the PID rate of its Defiance study, one of the Ten Investigator Prospective studies, was 15 to 20 times higher than the company had reported.

July 30–August 2, 1984: Roger Tuttle testifies in Minneapolis, claiming that A. H. Robins destroyed Dalkon Shield documents a decade earlier.

September–November 1984: A. H. Robins settles 198 Dalkon Shield cases with the Minnesota law firm of Robins, Zelle, Larson, and Kaplan for a record $38 million.

October 29, 1984: A. H. Robins announces its "removal program" for women still wearing the Dalkon Shield.

April 2, 1985
A. H. Robins announces it has set aside a reserve fund of $615 million to settle Dalkon Shield legal claims.

April 1985
The New England Journal of Medicine publishes results of two studies which directly link IUDs with infertility for the first time. According to the studies, the Dalkon Shield presents the greatest risk of infertility; its users have a three-to-seven-times-greater chance of becoming sterile than women who haven't worn the device.

Notes

During the course of the year it took us to research and write this book, we traveled from Washington, D.C., to Portland, Oregon, collecting thousands of pages of documents and interviewing more than 200 people. These travels included two journeys to the A. H. Robins Company headquarters in Richmond, Virginia, to talk with company officials. We have also attended some of the major court events of the past year: Judge Miles Lord's chastisement of the three A. H. Robins executives, Roger Tuttle's deposition, Lord's misconduct hearing, and the hearing concerning the removal and destruction of documents from the home of former A. H. Robins attorney Harris Wagenseil.

Because of the litigation that has surrounded the device for more than a decade, a staggering volume of material is available on the Dalkon Shield. Indeed, some of the key players in the Dalkon Shield story have given sworn testimony on the subject more than 50 times. In our attempt to get at the heart of this story, we have read thousands of pages of documents: internal A. H. Robins memos and correspondence; deposition and trial testimony of key players in the story; proceedings of various seminars, conferences, meetings, and congressional hearings; dozens of medical journal articles; and scores of newspaper and magazine articles published throughout the country. We also spent long hours collecting material from the National Medical Library in Bethesda, Maryland, and from the Food and Drug Administration's Freedom of Information Office, in nearby Rockville, Maryland.

Our major sourcebook for general medical information was the excellent book *Womancare*, by Lynda Madaras and Jane Patterson, M.D.

(Avon, 1981). For historical background on IUDs, Russel Thomsen's *An Atlas of Intrauterine Contraception* (Hemisphere Publishing, 1982) was invaluable. Government documents on which we heavily relied included the entire proceedings of the 1962 Intra-Uterine Contraceptive Devices Conference, the 1970 "Pill Hearings," the 1973 "Fountain Hearings" on the regulation of IUDs, and the 1975 "Kennedy Hearings" on FDA practices and procedures.

Index